The Phunny
Pharm

The Ultimate Pharmacology Study Guide

D1295257

The Phunny
Pharm

The Ultimate Pharmacology Study Guide

by

C. Ty Reidhead, MD

Department of Internal Medicine
University of Colorado Health Sciences Center
Denver, Colorado

with illustrations by

Michelle Van Santen

Hanley & Belfus, Inc./ Philadelphia
Mosby/ St. Louis • Baltimore • Boston • Carlsbad • Chicago • London
Madrid • Naples • New York • Philadelphia • Sydney • Tokyo • Toronto

Publisher: HANLEY & BELFUS, INC.
               210 South 13th Street
               Philadelphia, PA 19107
               (215) 546-7293
               FAX (215) 790-9330

North American and worldwide sales and distribution:

               MOSBY
               11830 Westline Industrial Drive
               St. Louis, MO 63146

In Canada: Times Mirror Professional Publishing, Ltd.
               130 Flaska Drive
               Markham, Ontario L6G 1B8
               Canada

Library of Congress Cataloging-in-Publication Data

Reidhead, C. Ty, 1968–
    The phunny pharm / C. Ty Reidhead.
        p.   cm.
    Includes index.
    ISBN 1-56053-114-2 (alk. paper)
    1. Drugs—Outlines, syllabi, etc.   2. Pharmacology—Outlines,
syllabi, etc.   3. Mnemonics.   I. Title.
    [DNLM: 1. Drugs—terminology.   2. Pharmacology—terminology.   QV
15 R359p 1996]
    RM301.14.R45   1996
    615′.1—dc20
    DNLM/DLC
    for Library of Congress   96-29285
                                                        CIP

The Phunny Pharm: The Ultimate Pharmacology Study Guide   ISBN 1-56053-114-2

Last digit is the print number: 9 8 7 6 5 4 3 2 1

Dedication

*To my wife, Mary, without whose support, encouragement, and sacrifice this book would
have remained "A regret that [I] did not begin."*

Table of Contents

Contributors vii
In Appreciation vii
Preface ix
Enter the Phunny Pharm 1
Phunny Pharm Anatomy by System 3
Antimicrobials—Sports
    Bacterial Name Guide 8
    Penicillins—Baseball 12
    Other Cell Wall Inhibitors 17
    Cephalosporins—Football 19
    Sulfonamides—Water Polo 23
    Tetracyclines—Cycling 26
    Broad-Spectrum Antibiotics—Basketball 28
    Aminoglycosides—Hockey 32
    Quinolones—Wrestling 35
    Antituberculosis Chemotherapy—Bobsledding 38
    Antifungals—Golf 41
    Antimalarial Chemotherapy—Pool 45
    Antiparasitics—Bowling 48
Antivirals and Antineoplastics—Dog Racing 53
    Antivirals—Dog Races and Viral Monsters 56
    Cancer Chemotherapy—Dog Races 62
The Autonomic Nervous System 71
    Parasympathetic Nervous System 76
    Parasympathomimetics:
        Things That Increase the Amount of Fish for the Bears and Cubs 78
    Parasympatholytics:
        Things That Decrease the Amount of Fish the Bears and Cubs Eat 83
    Neuromuscular Junction Blockers—NM Junction Gym 87
    Sympathetic Nervous System
    Sympathomimetics—Things That Scare Antelope, Vampires, and Bats 93
    Sympatholytics—Things That Control Antelope, Vampires, and Bats 99
Central Nervous System—The Phunny Pharm University 105
    Sedatives and Hypnotics—The University Pharm 106
    Anticonvulsants—Earthquake Prevention 113
    Antiparkinson's—Making the University Run 117
    Antipsychotics—The Crazy Library 122
    Drugs That Alter Mood—The MAO Fraternity 125
    Narcotic Analgesics—The University's Big-O Bar 130
Anesthesia 135
    General Anesthesia—The Airport and Planes That Bomb the University 135
    General Anesthesia Adjuncts 140
    Local Anesthetics—Shorting the Wires Monitoring Weather 143
Cardiovascular System—The Train and Roads of the Phunny Pharm 145
    Vasodilators—Enlarge Roads 148
    Diuretics—Cattle Drive Trail 155

Cardiac Inotropes—Stronger Train 160
Antiarrhythmics—Train Cars Interfering with the Engineers of the Train 164
Antihyperlipidemics—Fighting Crime... 172
Anticoagulation—Preventing or Removing Road Blocks 177
Inflammatory Mediators—Introduction 184
Nonsteroidal Antiinflammatory Drugs—Boats at the Beach 187
Antiulcers—Beach Damage Prevention.. 192
Antihistamines—Things That Eat Snakes in the Nose.. 196
Asthma—Keeping Airport Tubes Open.. 199
Index 205

Contributors

Contributing Author
Central Nervous System:
John P. Sheehan, MS IV

Illustrations
Michelle Van Santen

Creative Contributors*

Antimicrobials
John P. Sheehan, MS IV
Michael S. Sisk, MS IV
Sheri L. Drake, Veterinary Student yr. 3
Autonomic Nervous System
Michael S. Sisk, MS IV
John P. Sheehan, MS IV
Sheri L. Drake, Veterinary Student yr. 3
Cardiovascular System
William George, MS IV
Michael S. Sisk, MS IV

Antivirals and Cancer Chemotherapy
Michael S. Sisk, MS IV
Daniel O'Shea, Pre-Med

Central Nervous and Respiratory System
Michael S. Sisk, MS IV

Antiinflammatory and Gastrointestinal
John P. Sheehan, MS IV

Chapter Reviewers
David Arciniegas, M.D.
John Bisignano, M.D.
Thomas Elasy, M.D.
Andrea Iannucci, Pharm.D.
Ben Young, M.D., Ph.D.

In Appreciation
Thank you to Michelle Van Santen for your undying help in **years** that could have been much easier.

Thank you to John Sheehan and Mike Sisk for being there to help whenever I needed it and for helping me avoid the real Funny Farm.

Thank you to Frank Fitzpatrick, Ph.D., Linda Yardley, the late Charles Abernathy, M.D., Dean Nancy Nelson, M.D., and Robert Murphy, Ph.D., of the University of Colorado Health Sciences Center whose support was essential to *The Phunny Pharm*.

Thank you to my publisher, Linda Belfus, whose belief in a medical student she only briefly met will not be forgotten.

And finally, thank you to Trevor who sacrificed countless days in the park playing frisbee during work on *The Phunny Pharm*.

---

*The titles listed (MS IV, etc.) were true for the Creative Contributors when the book was being written.

"Just think . . . "

> Warren L. Reidhead, M.D. (<u>M</u>y <u>D</u>ad), and restated by
> Frank Fitzpatrick, Ph.D.

"They always said, 'A picture is worth a 1,000 words.' Who knew
that it would really take a 1,000 words to describe
the picture?!"

> John Sheehan, MS IV

Preface

On the somber day that we finally launched our study drive for Boards, we hauled out all of the syllabi that would be covered on the test and stacked them high to better visualize the task that lay before us. They towered above us ominously, so we quickly retreated to devise a plan for the next 2 weeks.

We easily saw weak links in the chain, such as classes that didn't teach us anything the first time around and were not about to help us now. This shortened the stack.

The next step was to consult with our elders. This was a very wise and valuable step, and with the advice of some friends, we disposed of everything but the big P.I.M.P.—Pharmacology, Immunology, Microbiology, and Pathology. Biochemistry was also important to study, but our syllabus was useless; reading a simple review book would be more efficient and effective than studying five pounds of syllabus.

We could only hope to knock the dust off of as much information in our meager minds in 2 weeks as possible. This meant getting through these subjects quickly and adequately.

Sounded easy at the time and sounds even easier now, but we weren't so lucky. We quickly discovered that as soon as we quit one topic, all of the newly reviewed information was lost. This was disturbing and scary, because we had time to get through all of these topics one time and one time only.

Pathology went by, then Micro, then Immuno, and then we moved on to Pharmacology. Pharm is a subject of abundant, minuscule, never-ending facts that seem impossible to retain. In our case, the syllabus alone was some 800 pages skinny, and to get through all of this in about 4 days was terrifying. Still, the only way to finish such a task was to begin.

The notebooks crept open at a discouraging pace, and we thumbed through to find the first section that we really needed to learn—the antimicrobials. Ahhh, there they were—the Sulfa drugs. "Okay: Time for a break. How about some breakfast and then we'll mow the lawn and vacuum the living room?" shouted someone from the other side of the table. There was one advantage of studying in a group—the others could motivate the slacker by threatening him with bodily harm or simply with falling behind.

In any case, we began without vacuuming, and much to our amazement, the antimicrobials were still fresh in our minds. Those first-learned facts were still in our brains, and, even more exciting, we could reinforce them with just a little practice. Unfortunately, after antimicrobials it was all downhill into dirt.

The only thing that we had done differently with the antimicrobials was to use pictures. Pictures that organized the drugs of each class in their proper place, where we would know exactly where to look. We had put each class on a different sport field, and all of the drugs were represented by a player on that field. All we had to do was picture that player and the field on which he played and we could recall everything that we needed to know. It was a heck of a lot easier than trying to remember which page that information had been on, what section, or, even worse, just to recall the facts from thin air.

Although it was not the photographic memory that I had always wanted, it was a way to use something that I already knew (i.e., sports) to learn something about which I knew absolutely nothing. Also, it was clear that everyone thinks in pictures, anyway. When someone says "dog," for example, one doesn't think of the letters d–o–g; instead, a clear image of a dog, probably growling or with a wagging tail, comes to mind. So, what better way of memorizing and retaining inordinate amounts of facts than to use images.

In this book, the pictures are already made and ready for review. I have taken many of the important facts I have learned and condensed the main points that are important for upcoming tests: the Boards, clerkships, and eventually practice of medicine.

Because every teacher's view of the important facts differs, the Phunny Pharm has been printed to allow room for additions to the pictures, new information as it becomes available, and doses that may be helpful to remember in internship and beyond. Finally, I have left room so that the pictures can be personalized, which will make them easier to remember.

Now that I have moved on to my clerkships, I realize that Pharmacology and Boards are not the only important times to remember drugs. In fact, a more important reason is that you will be prescribing drugs for the rest of your life and you begin to realize this importance when a resident asks about them. Believe me when I say there is nothing more frustrating than being asked for the **use** of a drug when you can't even put it in a **category.** This is the second purpose of this book—to provide a method of organization that will facilitate recall under the most unnerving circumstances and far into the future.

Please also remember that I intend this book only as a study aid. It is not intended as a guide to administration of medicines to patients.

C. Ty Reidhead

Enter the Phunny Pharm

The headlights dimmed, yielding to the glow of the city spreading out to the horizon, the music silenced, and the truck was filled with the piercing quiet of the desert. The ticking of the engine quickly invaded the stillness, and the quiet drone of the crickets in the distance reminded us that we were not alone.

I can picture this moment from my past like it happened yesterday. I do not remember the words to describe it, but the scene and the feelings that coursed through me remain vivid and easy to describe. This is simply because we think in pictures, not words or numbers. Because of this, it hurts my brain to remember information without anything with which to associate it. It is also why it seems easier to remember information during the third and fourth years of medical school, when we actually have patients with whom to associate the information.

Memorizing for the sake of memorization is not impossible as witnessed by the doctors that have made it through Pharmacology with this method. People have done this for years and will continue to do so in the future, but this does not have to be so.

The Phunny Pharm grew from this realization. It is a concept that we envisioned to bring order to the scattered information of Pharmacology. The Phunny Pharm actually represents the body, with each organ system represented by something that can be visualized within the Phunny Pharm. These systems are introduced in the Anatomy of the Phunny Pharm in Chapter 1. The Phunny Pharm then takes you through the drugs that affect each of the systems. Please don't worry about memorizing these now; you will become familiar with them as you go through the book.

    I. Antimicrobials—Sports
   II. Antiviral and Cancer Chemotherapy—Dog races
  III. Peripheral and Autonomic Nervous System—The Phunny Pharm Phorest
  IV. Central Nervous System—The university campus
   V. Anesthesia—The airport
  VI. Cardiovascular—A series of roads and a train that wind around the Phunny Pharm
 VII. Antiinflammatory—Boats
VIII. Gastrointestinal—Things on the beach and in the ocean
  IX. Asthma—Bats and the airport tubes

At the end of your journey through the Phunny Pharm, these systems will become second nature and you should have avoided being sent to the real Funny Farm.

Although you will likely develop your own approach, we offer a suggested approach for best results:

1. Begin by memorizing the Anatomy of the Phunny Pharm, as it contains associations that are used throughout the book.
2. Review the chapter to be covered prior to your lecture. Although you have heard this many times before, it would be awesome if you could leave your lectures in Pharmacology ready for the upcoming test and not have to review the material again.
3. Take *The Phunny Pharm* with you to class and take notes in it. Cross out the material you find extraneous, and add that which is not already in it.
4. Change the pictures to fit your needs.
5. If a picture doesn't work for you (not all of them will), skip the pictures and concentrate on the information.

Pictures do not magically remove the work involved in learning Pharmacology. Instead, they make it fun, more permanent, and enhance recall. This is important to remember because you may still find it difficult to get the information into your brain.

To enhance recall, practice recalling every point of each picture. When we learned the pictures for the antimicrobials, we were in a group of three. One person would recall aloud every piece of information in the picture he or she could visualize while the other two would check him and memorize the picture at the same time. Then we would switch and the next person would recall the picture for the other two. We would circle the table until every bit of information could be recalled without error. Although it is much easier in a group, this process can be done alone. Again recall the picture aloud and check yourself after you are done. Saying it aloud also reinforces the information, so don't be shy. Do this until you can recall the whole picture without error.

The most exciting part of the Phunny Pharm is the ability to hear a drug and place it into its class, so another exercise that may be worth practicing is to announce a drug to the group and have the others in the group place it in the proper picture. This should become easy with practice, as you will be able to recognize the drugs as a physical person or thing and then place it into the picture in which it belongs. Remember that all of this will take practice.

Phunny Pharm Anatomy by System

System

Analogy

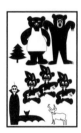
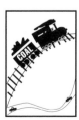

Antimicrobials
Antimicrobials
Microbes

Sports
Players of the sports
Opponents for the players

Central Nervous System
CNS toxicity

Phunny Pharm University
Things that can injure the Phunny
    Pharm University

Autonomic Nervous System
Parasympathetic nervous system
    Parasympathomimetic
    Parasympatholytic
Sympathetic nervous system

    Sympathomimetic

    Sympatholytic

Phunny Pharm Phorest
Nicky and her three musketeer cubs
    Actions of Nicky and the cubs
    Stopping the cubs
Nick the grizzly scaring antelope,
    vampires, and bats
    Actions of the antelope, vampires,
    and bats when they are scared
Stopping the antelope, vampires, or
bats

Respiratory
Lungs
Trachea, bronchi, bronchioles
Drugs that can be administered through
    the lungs
Respiratory secretions
Pulmonary toxicity

Phunny Pharm Airport
Airport
Tubes leading to the runways
All things that fly can use the airport
    to enter the Phunny Pharm
Rainstorms at the airport
Something is standing on a tube that
    leads to the Phunny Pharm Airport

Cardiovascular
Heart
    Inotropy
    Chronotropy
Arteries
Veins
Blood
Cardiovascular toxicity

Phunny Pharm Train
Train
    Strength of the train
    Speed of the train
Roads
Parking lots
Things that use the roads
Damage to the Phunny Pharm Train

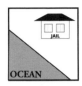

Gastrointestinal
Liver
Intestinal tract

Liver toxicity

Renal
Kidney

Secretions into the urine
Renal toxicity

Chemistry
Sodium
Calcium
Potassium
Protons/Hydrogen
Bicarbonate
Water

Ocean and Beach
Police station or jail
The ocean bordering the land of the
    Phunny Pharm
An injured jail or policeman

Shower at the End of the Trail
An "animal drive" in which cowboys
    are stealing animals from the
    Phunny Pharm. They are making
    their way to the shower at the end
    of the trail.
Anything that ends up in the shower
A broken shower

Steers
Calcium
Pigs
Hogs
Bees
Flies

Special Abbreviations
N	Name
mech	Mechanism of action
Dist	Distribution
Met	Metabolism
$t_{1/2}$	Half-life or duration of action
Tox	Toxicities and/or side effects
Rt	Route
Uses	Uses
R_x/R_x	Drug—drug interactions
→	Causes or yields
⇒	Implies
↑	Increase or makes larger
↓	Decrease or makes smaller
¢:	"Makes sense" and an explanation will usually follow it
Rem	Remember
CV	Cardiovascular
GI	Gastrointestinal

Antimicrobials—Sports

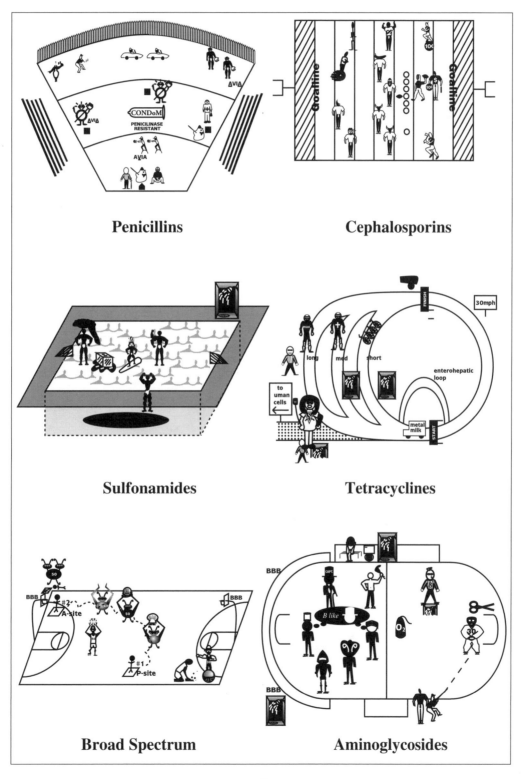

Penicillins

Cephalosporins

Sulfonamides

Tetracyclines

Broad Spectrum

Aminoglycosides

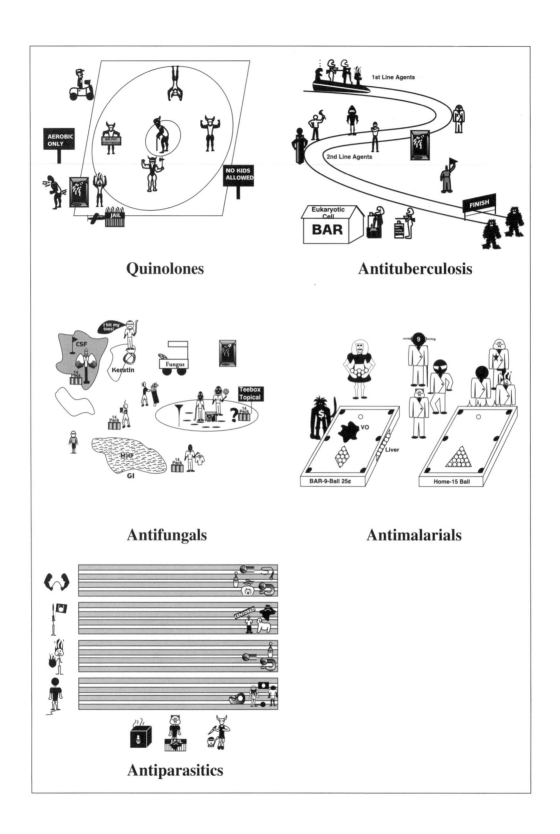

Quinolones

Antituberculosis

Antifungals

Antimalarials

Antiparasitics

Antimicrobials are fairly unique among pharmaceuticals because they are among the few medications capable of curing a disease. Diseases that are not surgically correctible are usually "treated," "suppressed," or "controlled," but not cured. Infectious diseases are an exception. With assistance from the patient's immune system, our great armamentarium of drugs provides an excellent prescription for a cure of most infections. Although these drugs can be rewarding to use, the prospect of learning to use them can be daunting to even an ambitious medical student.

From the original use of a sulfa drug in the 1930s and the mass production of penicillin in the 1940s, to the current list of well over 100 drugs, the number of antimicrobials has exploded. Although this growth largely reflects the scientific community's response to bacteria that have become harder to kill, it first left me dumbfounded and wondering where to begin. In *The Phunny Pharm*, we begin with the overall picture.

Picture Key

When the antimicrobials are separated into classes based on chemical structure and mechanism of action, they become much easier to learn. In this section of *The Phunny Pharm*, each class of antimicrobial has its own chapter, in which the antimicrobial class is represented by a sport, and the players in each sport represent the individual antimicrobials.

Penicillins	Baseball
Cephalosporins	Football
Sulfonamides	Water polo
Tetracyclines	Cycle races
Broad-spectrum antibiotics	Basketball
Aminoglycosides	Hockey
Quinolones	Wrestling
Antituberculosis chemotherapy	Bobsledding
Antimicrobials	Players in the respective sports
Microbes	Opponents the players are facing

Antimicrobial Uses

To make use of antimicrobials easier, try to follow these guidelines:

1. If you do not already have a firm grasp of the bugs that are common pathogens in humans, you should spend some time refreshing your memory.
2. Learn to place the antimicrobial in its general class (i.e., sport).
3. Learn the microbes for which the class of antimicrobial is used.
4. Try to learn the specific uses for each drug.
5. Finally, learn the microbes that cause the clinical syndromes, so empiric therapy can be chosen when an infection is suspected and the specific bug is not known*.

---

*There is no way around this once you get to the wards, even though you may not need to know this information for test purposes.

Bacterial Name Guide

Organism

Analogy

Gram-Positive Cocci

G$^+$ Cocci
Assoc
T$_x$ Penicillin
       First-generation cephalosporins

Baseball
G$^+$ Cocci look like baseballs
Baseball players
Defensive backs in the football game

Group <u>A</u> Streptococcus
Assoc
T$_x$ Penicillin G and V
       Other penicillins
       Cephalosporins
       Macrolides

The <u>G.A.S.</u> Baseball
First letters of the bacteria spell <u>gas</u>
The "captains" of the baseball players
Baseball players
Football players
Basketball players

Pneumococcus (*Strep. pneumoniae*)
Assoc
T$_x$ Penicillin G and V
       Penicillinase-resistant penicillins

       Cephalosporins
       Vancomycin in drug-resistant
          pneumococcus

New Moccasins
Sound alike
The captains of the baseball players
The infielders of the baseball game
    whose first letters spell CONDoM
Football players
Van the baseball catcher

Staphylococcus <u>a</u>ureus
Assoc

T$_x$ Penicillinase-resistant penicillins

       First-generation cephalosporins
       Erythromycin

       Vancomycin (2nd line)

Abominable <u>S</u>nowball
The first letters are the same, and <u>*S.*
aureus</u> is a monster bacteria
The infielders of the baseball game
    whose first letters spell CONDoM
Defensive backs of the football game
Free-throw mycin on the basketball
    team
Van the baseball catcher

Methicillin-<u>R</u>esistant
***Staphylococcus <u>a</u>ureus* (MRSA)**
Assoc   MRSA is tougher than *S. aureus*
T$_x$ Vancomycin
       Rifampin

<u>MR.</u> Abominable <u>S</u>nowball

MR. is MeaneR
Van the baseball catcher
Rifle man from the bob sledding

Enterococcus
Assoc   Sound alike
T$_x$ Gentamicin +
        Ampicillin

       Vancomycin

Terrible Cock

The gentleman hockey player
    The rightfielder from the baseball
       game
Van the baseball catcher

Gram-Negative Cocci

Neisseria <u>gonorrhoeae</u>

		Gondolas
Assoc		Gonorrhea sounds like gondola, and a gondola is where you could get gonorrhea.
T_x	Third-generation cephalosporins	The defense of the football game
	Spectinomycin	The young basketball player wearing spectacles
	Quinolones	Wrestlers

Neisseria <u>meningitidis</u>

		Nice Men in Tights
Assoc		Sound alike
T_x	Penicillin G	The captain of the baseball players
	Ceftriaxone	The running back of the football team

Gram-Negative Bacilli

G⁻ Bacillus

		Football
Assoc		Shaped like a football
T_x	Broad-spectrum penicillins	Amateur of right field in the baseball game
	Some second-generation cephalosporins, and all third-generation cephalosporins	The football players, especially the ones closest to the football
	Aminoglycosides	The hockey players

Escherichia coli

		Shrieking Collie
Assoc		Sound alike
T_x	≅ Anything that gets gram negatives:	
	Amoxicillin + β-lactamase inhibitor	Amateur of right field in the baseball game
	Cephalosporins	Football players
	Sulfamethoxazole/trimethoprim	Water polo player and goalie
	Aminoglycosides	Hockey players
	Fluoroquinolone	Wrestlers
	Nitrofurantoin	

Hemophilus <u>influenzae</u>

		Things that are <u>Insane</u>
Assoc		Sounds like "<u>one flew</u> over the cuckoo's nest" ⇒ insane
T_x	Amoxicillin and ampicillin	The baseball amateurs of right field
	Second and third-generation cephalosporins	The football defensive linemen and offense
	Sulfamethoxazole/trimethoprim	Water polo captain and goalie
	Fluoroquinolones	Wrestlers
	Second-generation macrolides	Basketball players

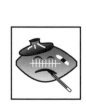

Pseudomonas aeruginosa

		Hypochondriac
Assoc		<u>Pseudomonas</u> ⇒ kind of + <u>monas</u> (sounds like <u>moaner</u>) ⇒ <u>kind of</u> + <u>moaner</u> = hypochondriac
T_x	Carbenicillin and ticarcillin	The centerfielders in the baseball game

Mezlocillin and piperacillin	The leftfielders in the baseball game
Imipenem	Rambocillin
Antipseudomonal third-generation cephalosporins	The offense in the football game
Antipseudomonal aminoglycosides	Hockey players

Klebsiella pneumoniae

A <u>Sale</u> on <u>Clubs</u>

Assoc

Klebs sounds like clubs

T_x	Ticarcillin + clavulanic acid	Centerfielder with the umpire
	Ampicillin + clavulanic acid	Amateur rightfielder with the umpire
	Third-generation cephalosporins	The offense of the football game
	Ciprofloxacin	Wrestler
	Antipseudomonal aminoglycosides	Hockey players

Enterobacter sp

The Bad <u>Emperor</u>

Assoc

Sound alike

T_x	Imipenem	Rambocillin
	Fluoroquinolones	Wrestler
	Sulfamethoxazole/Trimethoprim	Water polo captain and goalie

Moraxella catarrhalis

<u>Cat</u> with <u>More Axes</u>

Assoc

Sound alike

T_x	Amoxicillin and clavulanic acid	Amateur rightfielder with the umpire
	Carbenicillin and ticarcillin	The centerfielders in the baseball game
	Second- and third-generation cephalosporins	Defensive backs and linemen football players
	Sulfamethoxazole/trimethoprim	Basketball players
	Sulfamethoxazole/trimethoprim	Water polo player and goalie

Proteus mirabilis

<u>Proteus</u>

Assoc

Proteus was a Greek sea god who could assume different shapes.

| T_x | Ampicillin | Amateur of right field in the baseball game |
| | Sulfamethoxazole/trimethoprim | Water polo player and goalie |

Legionnella sp

<u>Legionnaire's</u> hat

Assoc

This is the hat that legionnaires wear.

| T_x | First- and second-generation macrolides | Part of the basketball team |
| | Sulfamethoxazole/trimethoprim | Water polo player and goalie |

Anaerobes

Bacteroides fragilis

The Hulk

Assoc	*B. fragilis* sounds like "fragile" but, in fact, this is a BAD bug	The Hulk is weak when human, but when he turns to the Hulk, he is a BAD dude.
T_x	Metronidazole	Volleyball coach
	Clindamycin	Clint the basketball coach
	Cefotetan, cefoxitin	Titan and Ox of the defensive line in the football game

Clostridium difficile

Assoc

T_x Metronidazole (PO)
         Vancomycin (PO)

Clothes on a Difficult Trident

Sound alike. The trident is alive.
Volleyball coach
Van the catcher

Atypicals

Mycoplasma pneumoniae

Assoc

T_x First- and second-generation
         macrolides
         Doxycycline

The Micro Plaid Man

Sound alike
Part of the basketball team

Cycler

Others

Chlamydia trachomatis

Assoc

T_x Tetracyclines (especially doxycycline)
         First- and second-generation macrolides
         Ofloxacin

Clam

Sound alike
Cyclers
Part of the basketball team
The old ox wrestler

Tuberculosis

Assoc   Tuberculosis
T_x First line:
             Isoniazid
             Rifampin
             Ethambutol
             Pyrazinamide
         Second line:
             Streptomycin
             p-Aminosalicylic acid
             Cycloserine

Bobsledder

Bobsledders compete in a Tube
In the bobsled:
    Ice on the Skid
    Rifle man
    Ethanol man
    Pyromaniac in the sled
On the track:
    The hockey player who strips
     PEZ candy man
    The psycho

Penicillins—Baseball

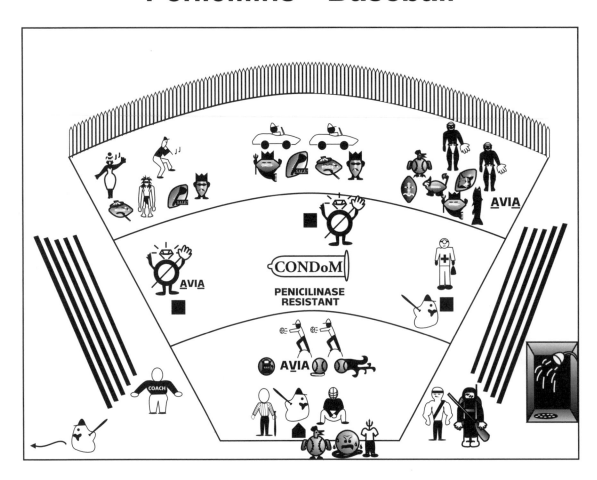

Picture Key

This is a baseball game in which the penicillins are on defense and the bacteria are at bat. The goal of the bacteria is to get on base and, of course, to score runs. Also, the bacteria have ways of protecting themselves from the defense. When the bacteria are at bat, they are attempting to cause an infection and the penicillins are stopping them.

Body	Baseball diamond
Penicillins	Defensive players on the field—the fielders
Bacteria	Opposing team—the batters
Penicillins at a therapeutic level	Player has to be on the field in order to fight the bacteria
Clavulanic acid	Umpire
β-lactamase	The bat that the bacteria use
Kidney	Sent to the showers*
Inflammation	The player is mad
Other cell wall inhibitors (similar mechanism of action, but are not penicillins) are also included in this chapter	The catcher, Rambo, and the astronaut with ammo

* Rem: Being sent to the showers represents metabolism by the kidney throughout *The Phunny Pharm*.

Penicillins in General

N	All end in -<u>cillin</u>	<u>Silly</u> baseball players
mech	<u>D-Ala-D-Ala</u> analogs	Players say "<u>eh-batta-eh-batta</u>."
	Covalent irreversible inhibition of <u>transpeptidase</u> in the synthesis of the cell wall	Players stop the <u>transit of the bases</u> by the bacteria.
Dist	Penetrates <u>inflamed</u> tissues more readily	Players try harder when they are mad.
Met	Excreted unchanged in urine	Sent to the showers
	Secreted by renal tubules	
$t_{1/2}$	<1 hr	
Tox	See below	The baseball fan
Rt	IM rapid absorption; can use insoluble <u>salts</u> to reduce absorption rate	If the players are eating <u>salty</u> sunflower seeds, they will go into the game after they are through, thereby saving some of the players for later in the game
	PO need much higher dose, some are absorbed better than others, and oral penicillins are acid-resistant	The players that can be taken PO, spell AVIA. AVIA also is a shoe brand that protects their feet from acid ⇒ acid-resistant.
Uses	G^+	Because the game is baseball, the players are best against a <u>baseball</u>.
Res	<u>β-lactamase</u>—plasmid-mediated	Batters have the <u>bat</u> and try to carry it around the bases with them so they can protect themselves from the penicillins.
	This plamid can be transferred to other bacteria.	The bat can be handed to the next batter.
	Escape	If the competition is too tough, the batter can escape.

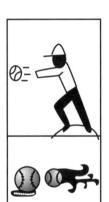

	Penicillin G and Penicillin V	**The Pitchers**
N	Penicillin G	The pitchers of the team
	Penicillin V (essentially oral penicillin G)	
Rt	IM or IV	Muscular
	PO for penicillin <u>V</u>	Part of AVIA
Uses	<u>Group A</u> Strep	Throw fastballs and try to light the <u>G.A.S.</u> ball on fire—trying to "smoke 'em"
	<u>Pneumococci</u> and many others	They really try to get batters with the <u>new moccasins</u>

Penicillinase-Resistant Penicillins   The Infielders

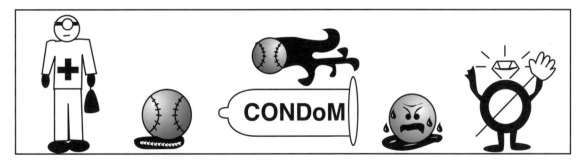

	DOCs	**Not Married**
N	<u>C</u>loxacillin, <u>O</u>xacillin, <u>N</u>afcillin, <u>D</u>icloxacillin, <u>M</u>ethicillin	First letters spell <u>CONDoM</u>.

Isoxazoles end in -oxacillin: / The mouth <u>DOC</u>s on first base of the infield

<u>Di</u>cloxacillin, <u>O</u>xacillin, and <u>C</u>loxacillin / Infielders who are <u>not</u> <u>m</u>arried—the

<u>Na</u>fcillin and <u>M</u>ethicillin / second and third basemen

mech Resistant to β-<u>lactamase</u> / The <u>COND</u>o<u>M</u> protects them from the <u>bat.</u>

Rt Isoxazoles are PO / Isoxazole is part of AV<u>I</u>A ⇒ acid-resistant

<u>Na</u>fcillin and <u>M</u>ethicillin are parenteral / Not part of AVIA ⇒ parenteral

Uses Penicillinase-producing <u>Staphylococcus</u> / When the pitcher cannot strike out the batter, then the infielders would love to get him, especially the Abominable Snowball.

<u>Pneumococci</u> / They really try to get the batters with the <u>new moccasins</u>.

Group <u>A</u> Strep / They also like to burn the <u>G.A.S.</u> man.

Res If bacteria is resistant to these drugs, then the bacteria is "methicillin-resistant" (e.g., Methicillin-Resistant *S. aureus* ≡ MRSA) / This is an important point to remember for wards.

Extended-Spectrum Penicillins   The Outfielders

N <u>Amp</u>icillin, <u>Amo</u>xicillin, / The <u>am</u>ateur rightfielders

<u>C</u>arbenicillin, <u>Ti</u>carcillin, / The <u>c</u>en<u>t</u>erfielders

<u>Me</u>zlocillin, <u>P</u>iperacillin / The <u>le</u>ftfielders

Uses Extended spectrum / Outfielders cover a larger area

Ampicillin and Amoxicillin   **Amateur Rightfielders**

N <u>Amp</u>icillin / The right field is where the least number of balls are hit, so the <u>am</u>ateurs play right field.

<u>Amo</u>xicillin

Rt PO / Both are part of AV<u>IA</u> ⇒ acid-resistant.

Uses Same as for Pen G as well as others: / Since they are the young players on the team, they look up to the pitcher.

<u>Prote</u>us / They like to get the sea god <u>Prote</u>us.

E. coli / They love to play with the <u>shrieking collie</u>.

H. in<u>flu</u>enzae / They hit the <u>insane</u> bacteria.

Enterococcus / Not afraid of the <u>terrible cock</u>

Moraxella <u>cat</u>arrhalis / Take the <u>ax</u> from the <u>cat</u>.

R$_x$/R$_x$ Decrease birth control pill effectiveness → pregnancy / Because they are so young, they do not know how to prevent pregnancy.

Antipseudomonal Penicillins

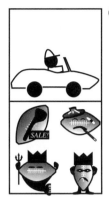

Carbenicillin and Ticarcillin

N	Carbenicillin
	Ticarcillin
Rt	Parenteral
Uses	Pseudomonas
	Proteus
	Enterobacter
	Klebsiella

The Centerfielder in the Car

The centerfielder has to cover such a large area of the field, so he drives a car.

Not part of AVIA
They like to run over hypochondriacs.
They like to run over Proteus.
They like to run over the bad emperor.
They like to run over the sale on clubs.

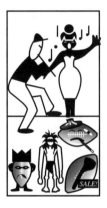

Mezlocillin and Piperacillin

N	Mezlocillin
	Piperacillin
Rt	Parenteral
Uses	*Klebsiella pneumoniae*
	Bacteroides fragilis
	Pseudomonas
	Enterobacter

The Musicians of Left Field

The leftfielders are a "mezzo"*
and a piper.
Not part of AVIA
They like to get the clubs on sale.
They like to get the Hulk.[†]
They like to run over hypochondriacs.
They like to run over the bad emperor.

Penicillin Toxicity

Allergic reaction $\Rightarrow$ from rash to anaphylaxis
Seizures
Na^+ and K^+ intoxication with parenteral use of Antipseudomonal penicillins

The Baseball Fan

He has a rash and passes out.

The fan will have problems if he injects steers and pigs[‡] instead of eating them.

---

*Mezzo is a Soprano.
[†]Rem: The Hulk is a guy who appears to be fragile but is really the ferocious Hulk. This is similar to *fragilis* because the name would imply a wimpy bug, when in fact this is a Bad Bug.
[‡]Rem: From the diuretics chapter, sodium $\Rightarrow$ steers and potassium $\Rightarrow$ pigs.

Adjuncts to Penicillins

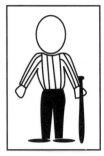

Clavulanate, Sulbactam, Tazobactam

mech   No antibacterial activity, but inhibit β-lactamase

Uses   Clavulanate + ticarcillin to make Timentin (Beecham Labs, Bristol, IN)

Clavulanate + amoxicillin to make Augmentin (Beecham Labs, Bristol, IN)

Piperacillin + tazobactam to make Zosyn* (Lederle Piperacillin, Pearl River, NY)

The Umpires

The umpires can take the bat away from the batters.

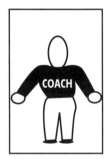

Probenicid

mech   No antibacterial activity, but inhibits renal secretion of penicillins ⇒ prolongs $t_{1/2}$

The Coach Probes the Field

Keeps the players from going to the showers, so they remain on the field longer.

---

*This combination should not be used for *Pseudomonas,* because the formulation does not allow for adequate doses of piperacillin for *Pseudomonas.*

Other Cell Wall Inhibitors

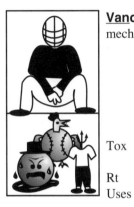

Vancomycin

mech	Inhibits assembly of cell wall by inhibition of peptidoglycan polymers transport to cell wall; this occurs at a different step than β-lactamases
	Resistant to β-lactamases; also not affected by methicillin resistance
Tox	<u>Red</u> man's syndrome with rapid IV administration
Rt	<u>IV</u>
Uses	Penicillin resistance: Even though vancomycin will get strep and staph that are resistant to penicillin, β-lactamase-resistant penicillins are more efficacious
	MRSA
	Clostridium difficile used PO
	Enterococcus

Van the Catcher

Hits the batter as he is walking to the batter's box (i.e., <u>before</u> he can transit the bases)

Padding protects him from the bat that the batters carry

Gets red with <u>embarrassment</u> when he has to put on his <u>ivory</u> helmet

Wears an <u>ivory</u> helmet

If the batter gets all the way around the bases and no one got him out, then the catcher will get him before the batter makes a run.

If the batter is <u>MR. Abominable Snowball,</u> then the catcher just takes him out of the game before he can bat.

Hits the <u>difficult</u> <u>trident</u> in <u>clothes</u>

Hits the <u>terrible cock</u>

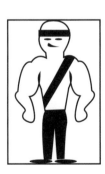

Imipenem

N	Imipenem
mech	β-Lactamase that inhibits crosslinking of cell wall components
Uses	With cilastatin, which inhibits the renal metabolism of imipenem
	Has the broadest antibacterial spectrum

Rambocillin

Although the relation to Rambocillin is not obvious, it is easy to remember when you consider there is very little resistance to it and that it has a very broad spectrum.

Rambo can kill just about any bacteria.

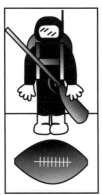

Aztreonam

mech   β-lactamase

Uses   Gram-negative coverage without the side effect of hypersensitivity seen with penicillins

Pseudomonas aeruginosa

Not used for anaerobes or <u>gram-positives</u>

The <u>Astro</u>naut with <u>Ammo</u>

The ammunition (ammo) that the astronaut has is special, so that it only gets football players, and the space suit keeps the patient's body from becoming allergic to the astronaut.

The ammo destroys the <u>hypo-chondriac</u>*.

The ammo does not work for the <u>baseballs</u>.

---

*Rem: Hypochondriacs = *Pseudomonas* because *Pseudomonas* sounds like "pseudo + moaner."

Cephalosporins—Football

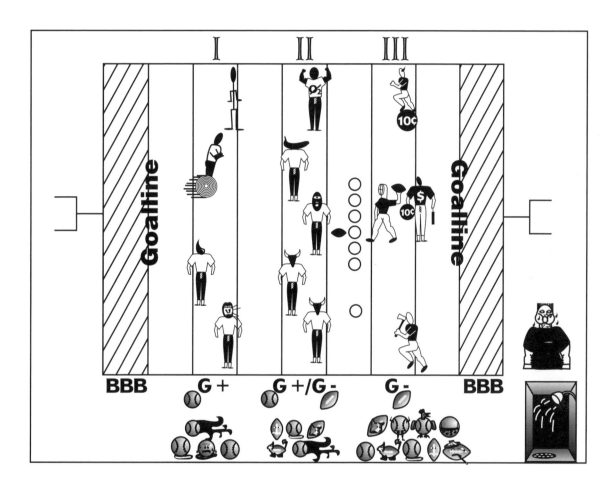

Picture Key

In this picture, the cephalosporins are football players and their positions on the field help to keep straight the three generations of cephalosporins. Bacteria in this picture are not competing <u>against</u> the cephalosporins, but do appear in the picture.

Blood–brain barrier (BBB)	Goal line
To cross BBB	To make a touchdown
If inflammation is present	A player has made an interception
First generation	Defensive backs
Second generation	Defensive linemen
Third generation	Offense
Activity against G⁻ bacteria	The proximity to the football
Kidney	The showers
Liver	Referee

Cephalosporins in General

N	All begin with the sound "cef-" except moxalactam	
mech	Inhibition of cell wall synthesis in same manner as penicillins (i.e. β-lactams) ⇒ inhibit <u>transpeptidase</u>	Just remember that the football players work in the same fashion as the baseball players ⇒ stop the "<u>transit of bases</u>."
	They are bactericidal	
Dist	Only third generation can cross BBB	Only generation that is on offense and can make a touchdown
Met	Primarily secreted by the <u>kidney</u>	Players can go to the <u>showers</u> after the game.
Tox	See picture of football fan below	The football fan
Rt	All are IV and IM unless indicated in the picture	
Uses	First generation ⇒ G$^+$ mainly	The defensive backs are furthest from the football.
	Second generation ⇒ G$^+$ and G$^-$	The defensive linemen are close to the football, but the offense has the ball; therefore, the offense is "closest" to the football and gets the most G$^-$.*
	Third generation ⇒ G$^-$ mainly	

First Generation (I)   Defensive Backs

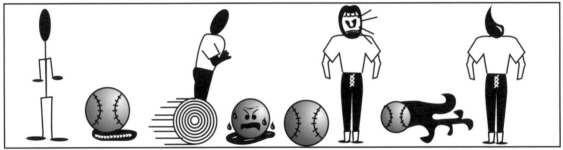

	Cephalothin Cefazolin	Cephalexin Cefadroxil
N	Cephalo<u>thin</u>	This defensive back is <u>thin</u>.
	Cefa<u>zolin</u>	Once he gets <u>rollin'</u> he can run fast.
	Cepha<u>lexin</u>	He let a receiver make a touchdown so he got <u>lectured</u>.
	Cefa<u>droxil</u>	<u>Dropped</u> an interception
Dist	Can't cross the BBB except when it is inflamed	Defensive backs can only make a touchdown if they intercept the football.
$t_{1/2}$	Cephalothin has a <u>shorter</u> $t_{1/2}$ than other first generations	Because he is thin, he <u>retires to the showers earlier</u> than other defensive backs.
Rt	Cephalothin is by IV only	Because he is so thin, there is not enough muscle to inject into, and he doesn't eat.
	Cephalexin is <u>PO</u>	Cephalexin got lectured, which is done by the <u>mouth</u>.
Uses	Good activity vs. <u>G</u>$^+$ bacteria and little activity vs. <u>G</u>$^-$	Love to tackle the bacteria that play <u>baseball</u>. They are also furthest away from the <u>football</u>* when lined up ⇒ they have the least activity vs. G$^-$.
	<u>Pneumococcus</u> (*Streptococcus pneumoniae*)	Defensive backs like to tackle the team with the <u>new moccasins</u>.
	<u>G</u>roup <u>A</u> <u>S</u>trep	Defensive backs like to tackle the GAS baseball.
	<u>S</u>taphylococcus <u>a</u>ureus	Defensive backs like to tackle the <u>A</u>bominable <u>S</u>nowball.

*Rem: Bacterial <u>Baseball</u> players ⇒ <u>G</u>$^+$ cocci and bacterial <u>football</u> players ⇒ G$^-$ bacilli.

Second Generation (II)   Defensive Line

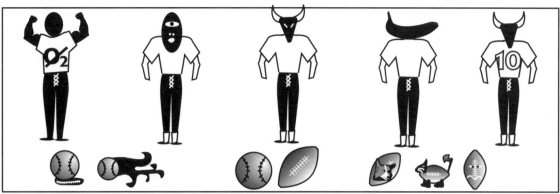

| | Cefotetan | Cefaclor | Cefuroxime | Cefamandole | Cefoxitin |

N   Begin in Cef-   They are the defensive line; they have to be
                                                            big guys

       otetan   The <u>titan</u>

       aclor   The cyclops named <u>Clor</u>

       uroxime   The <u>furious ox</u>

       amandole   The <u>maniac</u> who likes <u>dole</u> bananas.

       oxitin   The <u>ox</u> who is <u>#10</u>.

Rt   Cefotetan is IM only   This titan is very <u>muscular</u>.

      Cefa<u>clor</u> is PO   <u>Clor</u> sounds like <u>oral</u>.

Uses   They cover more G⁺ than the first generation and   Closer to football in the line-up
            therefore are good agents for community-
            acquired upper respiratory infections and
            pneumonias.

      *H. influ*enzae   They like to get the players from the <u>insane
                                                            asylum</u>.

      <u>G</u>roup <u>A</u> <u>S</u>trep   They tackle the <u>GAS</u> baseball.

      <u>Pneu</u>mococcus (*Streptococcus pneumoniae*)   Defensive linemen tackle the team with the
                                                            <u>new moccasins</u>.

      Moraxella catarrhalis   Defensive linemen strip the <u>cat</u> with <u>more
                                                            axes</u>.

      Escherichia coli   Defensive linemen get the <u>shrieking collie</u>.

Third Generation (III)   Offense

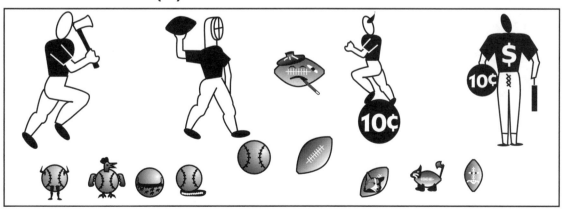

| Ceftriaxone | Cefoperazone | Ceftazidime | Cefotaxime |

N	End in -<u>zone</u> ⇒ Cef____one	They end in the sound "zone" ⇒ can get into end<u>zone</u>.
	Cef<u>tri</u>a<u>x</u>one	The running back <u>tries</u> to <u>ax</u> his way through the defense and to the end <u>zone</u>.
	Cefo<u>pera</u>zone	The quarterback needs a <u>peri</u>scoping neck in order to see the field and get into the end <u>zone</u>.
	End in -ime ⇒ Cef____ime	
	Cef<u>tazi</u>dime	This running back is a <u>Tazmanian Devil</u> who turns on a <u>dime</u>.
	Cefo<u>taxi</u>me	The <u>tax</u> man who keeps the <u>dime</u> on which he turns
Met	Cefoperazone is mainly <u>hepatic</u>—into bile	He is bothered most by the <u>referee</u>* because he is the leader of the team.
Dist	<u>BBB</u> does not have to be inflamed in order to cross	Offense does not have to make an interception before they can get into the <u>endzone</u>
Uses	They mainly cover G⁻ bacilli	They have the football† and are therefore as close as the drugs can get to the football.
	Neisseria <u>gonorrhea</u>	The offense smashes the <u>gondola</u> team.
	Neisseria <u>meningitidis</u>	The offense smashes the <u>nice men in tights</u>.
	<u>Escherichia coli</u>	The offense smashes the <u>shrieking collie</u>.
	H. <u>influenzae</u>	The offense smashes <u>insane</u> football players‡
	<u>Moraxella</u> <u>catarrhalis</u>	The offense smashes the <u>cat</u> with <u>more axes</u>.
	Also get some G⁺ bacilli	The offense will get some baseball players.
	<u>Enterococcus</u>	They smash the <u>terrible cock</u>.
	<u>Pneumococcus</u> (*Streptococcus pneumoniae*)	The offense smashes the team with <u>new moccasins</u>.
	Cefoperazone and ceftazidime cover *<u>Pseudomonas</u> aeruginosa*	The quarterback with the parascoping neck and the Tazmanian Devil who turns on a dime smash hypochondriacs.§

Cephalosporin Toxicity

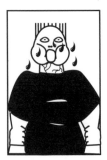

Sensitivity
Thrombophlebitis
Disulfuram-like reaction
Neurotoxicity

The Fan

Cries very easily if his team loses
Neck veins are sticking out
Drinks EtOH and is vomiting
Does not like college teams, only professional¶

---

*Rem: The referee is the liver in this picture.
†Rem: Football shaped like a bacillus.
‡Rem: <u>Haemophilus influenzae</u> is represented by things that are insane, because influenza sounds like "One flew over the cuckoo's nest."
§Rem: Hypochondriacs = <u>Pseudomonas</u> because <u>Pseudomonas</u> sounds like "pseudo + moaner."
¶Rem: University signifies the CNS throughout the Phunny Pharm.

Sulfonamides—Water Polo

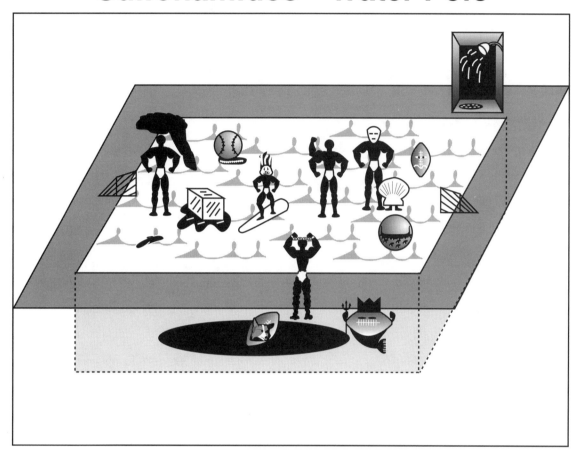

Picture Key

This is a picture of a water polo game in which the sulfonamides are trying to score a goal on the bacteria, who are on the other team. Because water solubility is an important issue in the sulfonamides, this is represented by the ability of the players to swim or at least remain afloat.

Sulfonamides	Water polo players
The human body	Swimming pool
Kidney	The drain
Liver	Referee
Water solubility	The ability of player to swim or remain afloat
Proteins in the blood	H_2O wings
Trimethoprim	Goalie of the sulfonamide team

Sulfonamides in General

N   All begin with sulfa-

mech   Bacteriostatic   Not a rough sport and they are just trying to stop the opposing team, not kill them

PABA analogs = inhibits dihydropteroate synthase, important in folate synthesis

Dist   Weak acid
       Extensive protein binding

All water polo players like to use H$_2$O wings ⇒ helps them remain afloat.

Met   Hepatic ⇒ N-acetylation → decreased solubility of the sulfonamide

Handcuffs placed on the water polo players by the referee inhibit the players' ability to swim.

Tox   Crystalluria

Players may plug the drain.

       Rash (Stevens Johnson syndrome) with long acting

If in H$_2$O too long ⇒ get wrinkled

       Hemolytic anemia in G6PD

       Kernicterus in neonates 2° to protein displacement of bilirubin

Limited number of H$_2$O wings—none left for kids, so they become yellow with envy

R$_x$/R$_x$ Displacement of other R$_x$s from circulating proteins; a good example is coumadin → increased anticoagulation

No H$_2$O wings left for other R$_x$s.

Uses   Bacterial resistance limits its usefulness, but still covers a broad spectrum

       Mainly used with trimethoprim ⇒ Bactrim for sinusitis, otitis media, and urinary tract infections

Water polo players mainly play when goalie is around. Will clean the drain* if blocked by opponents

       Bacteria covered:

The water polo players, with the goalie, drown

          Hemophilus influenzae

The insane swimmers

          Escherichia coli

The shrieking collie, who can't swim anyhow

          Proteus

Proteus the Greek sea god made a mistake and changes himself into a rock that cannot swim

          Legionella

The old legionnaire who can't swim, so he is an easy target for them

          Pneumocystis carinii

          Pneumococcus (*Strep. pneumonia*)

When the new moccasins are wet they are too heavy with which to swim.

          Gonorrhea

They like to beat the team cheating with gondolas.

Triple Sulfas: Sulfadiazine, Sulfamerazine, Sulfamethazine

N   Sulfa_____azine
      di
      mer
      meth

Uses   Used together ⇒ the advantage is that solubilities are independent of other two drugs, but actions are additive

Sulfa Di-Mer-Methazine—A Water Polo Player with Three Arms

Sulfa Di-Mer-Methazine

Three arms help to swim better and can also play better.

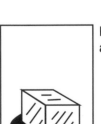

More Soluble Sulfas: Sulfisoxazole and Sulfamethoxazole

N   Sulf_____oxazole
      iso
      ameth

Mech   More soluble than other sulfas, so they don't cause as much crystallinuria

Ice and a Mess Float on Water

"Ice" floats on H$_2$O
but makes a mess.
Things that float on water

---

*Note: This is the only place in The Phunny Pharm where the kidney is not represented by a shower.

Topical Sulfas

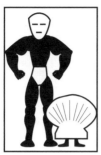

Sulfacetamide
Use   Ophthalmic only
      Chlamydia trachomatis in
        conjunctival cells

Wearing "**Face**" Mask
Face mask protects <u>eyes.</u>
The mask protects him from the clam.

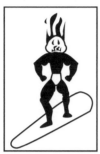

Silver Sulfadiazine
Use   <u>Burns</u>

Silver Surfer
The Silver Surfer's hair is on <u>fire.</u>

Sulfonamide Synergists

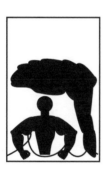

Trimethoprim
N   <u>Trimethoprim</u>

Mech   Inhibits <u>dihydrofolate</u> <u>reductase</u>

Use   Synergism with sulfas

Tries Methane Primarily
<u>Tries</u> <u>meth</u>ane <u>pri</u>marily to make a smoke
    screen and help him protect the goal
Reduces the dying H_2O foliage by
    burning it
He is the goalie of the Sulfa team and
    therefore works together with the sulfas
    to beat the bacteria.

Tetracyclines—Cycling

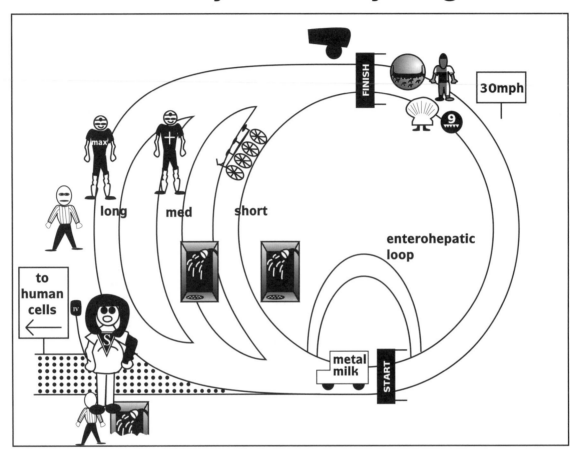

Picture Key

This picture is of a bicycle track in which there are three loops to the track. The tetracyclines are represented by the bicycles and the bacteria are the finish line. The goal is to get the cycles to the bacteria so that they can do their stuff.

Tetracyclines	Cycles on the various tracks of the race course
Renal excretion	Showers on the tracks where renal metabolism occurs
Toxicity	The cycle superfan
Entrance into body	Start line
Bacteria	Finish line

Tetracyclines in General

N	End in -cycline	Sounds like bicycling
mech	30s Ribosome	Speed limit 30 mph sign
	Uptake into bacteria is active and passive.	
Met	Kidney and liver	There are showers and referees on the track:
	Short and intermediate tetracyclines are mainly by kidney.	There are showers on the short and medium loops of the track.
	All are partially excreted in bile and reabsorbed.	The enterohepatic loop located at the start of the track

26

	Tetracyclines can get into mammalian cells but not as easily as they do into the bacteria.	Dirt road leads to the mammalian cells. Via this road, the cycles can get to the mammalian cells, but it is harder to ride on than the other road.
$t_{1/2}$	Grouped into long, intermediate, and short	There are three different loops on the track.
Tox	Summarized below	See the superfan
Rt	Orally available but absorption impaired by <u>metal ions</u> and <u>milk</u>	<u>Metal milk truck</u> at the start line that blocks the road and prevents the cycles from racing around the track
Uses	Broad spectrum	Bacteria that are sitting at the finish line and will be run over by the cycles:
	Malaria	The mean nine ball*
	Chlamydia trachomatis	A <u>clam</u>
	Mycoplasma pneumoniae	The <u>micro plaid man</u>
	Amebiasis	
Res	Resistance is by <u>decreased uptake</u> and	Bacteria can put up a <u>road block</u> at finish line, making it more difficult to get to it.
	<u>Active transport out</u> of cell	<u>Cannon</u> at finish line that shoots cycles back to start line.

Tetracyclines   # Cyclists

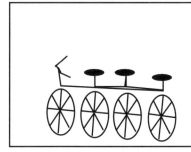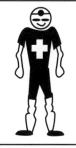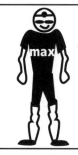

Tetracycline   **Methacycline and   **Minocycline and
                          Demeclocycline**   Doxycycline**

N	<u>Tetra</u>cycline	A <u>four</u>-wheeled cycle
	<u>M</u>ethacycline and <u>D</u>emeclocycline	First letters of names spell <u>M.D.</u>
	<u>M</u>inocycline and <u>D</u>oxycycline	<u>Max</u>imum length <u>drug</u>
$t_{1/2}$	Short $t_{1/2}$ ⇒ <u>Tetra</u>cycline	Represent the tracks they ride on
	Medium $t_{1/2}$ ⇒ <u>M</u>ethacycline and <u>D</u>emeclocycline	
	Long $t_{1/2}$ ⇒ <u>M</u>inocycline and <u>D</u>oxycycline	

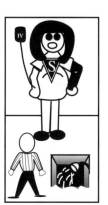

Tetracycline Toxicity   **The Superfan**

<u>Super</u>infection ⇒ tetracyclines kill normal flora of the bowel so they can no longer inhibit the growth of more toxic flora	<u>Super</u>fan
Hepatotoxicity	The superfan never agrees with the referee and she yells at him until he is sick.
Contraindicated in pregnancy and in children up to 8 yr because of bone and teeth effects	She's pregnant.
Bone and teeth effects: <u>Staining</u> and maldevelopment	A cast is on her arm: It is a <u>black</u> cast (i.e., it was stained).
Coagulopathy—vitamin K deficiency	IV bottle ⇒ signifying replacement
<u>Renal</u> toxicity	She broke the showers.
Photosensitivity	She is wearing sunglasses.

*The mean nine ball is malaria, as will be seen in the chapter on malaria.

Broad-Spectrum Antibiotics—Basketball

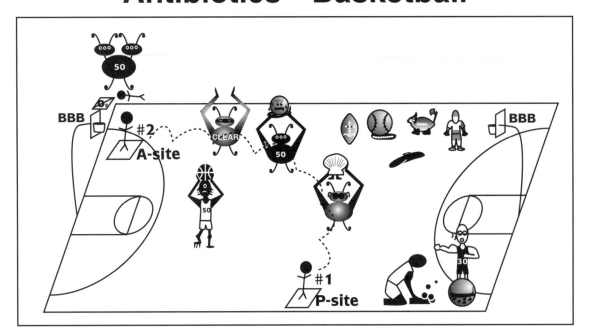

Picture Key

This is a picture of a basketball game in which the broad-spectrum antibiotics are playing the bacteria. The bacteria move the ball down court and score, while the broad-spectrum antibiotics try to stop them. Because these antibiotics work by blocking protein synthesis, the antibiotics are seen stealing the ball from the bacteria at different places on the court. Please note that the opposing players represent the bacteria and the bacterial ribosome with which the antibiotic interferes.

Broad-spectrum antibiotics	Basketball players
Bacteria	Opposing team players
Bacterial ribosome	Opposing team players
Protein synthesis	Movement of ball down the court
Protein made by the ribosome	The basketball the players are passing along
30s ribosome	Young basketball player—only 30 years old
50s ribosome	Old basketball player—50 years old
Crosses blood–brain barrier (BBB)	The basketball player can slam dunk.
Court	Cell membrane
Kidney	The showers in the locker room
Liver	The referee

Review of Protein Synthesis—Movement of Ball Down Court

1. t-RNA with protein already in P-site

    Player #1 has the ball and is ready to make a basket; but he must wait until another player is under the basket to rebound the ball.

2. t-RNA enters A-site

    Player #2 goes to a site where he can rebound the shot at the basket ⟹ the Acceptor-site.

28

3. Peptidyl transferase <u>moves protein chain</u> onto amino acid of t-RNA in <u>A</u>-site

Player #1 <u>shoots the ball</u> at the basket and player #2, who is at the <u>acceptor</u>-site, catches the ball.

4. Translocation ⇒ t-RNA in A-site is <u>moved</u> into P-site

Player #2 <u>dribbles</u> the ball to the P-site and prepares to take another shot when a new player enters the A-site.

Broad-Spectrum Antibiotics in General

Mech   Bacterio<u>static</u>

Basketball is supposed to be a noncontact sport: They do not try to kill the opponents; just stop them.

         Block protein synthesis

Keeps other team from moving ball down the court

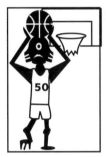

Chloramphenicol
mech   <u>50s</u> ribosome

A <u>Cyclops, Amphibian</u>
One of the <u>old</u> guys" ⇒ he is 50 years old

      Blocks peptidyl transferase reaction

He blocks the shot at the basket.

Dist   Crosses BBB

Can slam dunk ⇒ great for an older player

Met   Conjugated to glucuronide or excreted unchanged by the <u>kidney</u>

Referee <u>glues</u> him to the floor or he is sent to the showers.

Tox   Bone marrow suppression

Can get <u>dried bones</u>.* Because he is an amphibian, he dries out if he is out of H_2O too long.

      Blood dyscrasias
      Hemolytic anemia in G6PD deficiency
      More reports of the following than with other antibiotics:
      Fatal aplastic anemia
      Superinfections—*Clostridium difficile* colitis →
      <u>Pseudomembr</u>anous colitis

He doesn't get to play anymore ⇒ kind of (i.e., <u>pseudo</u>) <u>a member</u> of the team.

      Infants—gray baby syndrome

His babies are gray because born in H_2O.

R_x/R_x Inhibits cytochrome P-450
Uses   Infections where other antibiotics are ineffective or contraindicated because of the seriousness of the side effects

Only comes into game when he is needed

---

*Rem: Dry bones ⇒ bone marrow suppression.

Macrolides

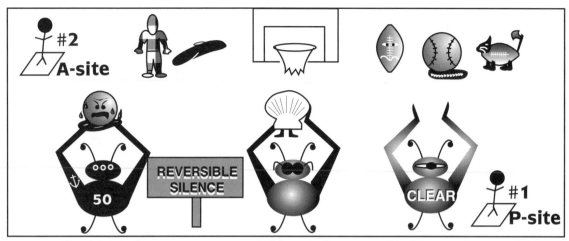

	Erythromycin	**Azithromycin**	**Clarithromycin**
N	Erythromycin Azithromycin Clarithromycin	Free-throw mycin—a martian Amazing-throw mycin Clear-the-throw mycin	
mech	50s ribosome Blocks translocation from A- to P-site	He is one of the "old guys." They steal the ball from the dribbler when he tries to move the ball back outside for another shot (i.e., before the P-site).	
Met	1° by liver Erythromycin is concentrated and secreted in bile	Ejected from the game by referee Free throw is a green man (a martian)—bile is green.	
Tox	Nausea, vomiting, and diarrhea Erythromycin → Hepatotoxicity Erythromycin and Azithromycin → Reversible hearing loss Azithromycin → photosensitivity	 Free throw freezes the referee. Free throw and Amazing have a sign between them that reads, "Reversible Silence." Amazing is wearing sunglasses.	
R_x/R_x	Inhibit cytochrome P-450		
Uses	Legionella Mycoplasma *Moraxella catarrhalis* Pneumococcus (*Streptococcus pneumoniae*) *Hemophilus influenzae* Azithromycin ⇒ single dose for chlamydia Erythromycin ⇒ *Staphylococcus aureus*	They stop the legionnaire. They stop the micro plaid man. They stop the cat with more axes. They stop the player wearing the new moccasins. They stop the insane player. Amazing can stop the clam. Free throw can stop the Abominable Snowball.	

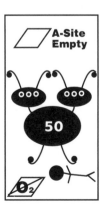

	Clindamycin and Lincomycin	**Siamese Twin Coaches ⇒ Clint and Link (Linked to Clint)**
mech	50s ribosome Block attachment of t-RNA to ribosome—m-RNA complex	They are "old guys." Knocks player out before he can get to the A-site (i.e., when he is coming into the game)
Rt	PO or IV	The coach does a lot of yelling.
Met	1° by liver Concentrated and secreted in bile	Gets thrown out by referee Green man—he is also a martian
Tox	Pseudomembranous colitis	Coach ⇒ kind of (i.e., pseudo) a member of the team
Uses	Staph infections where penicillin not indicated Anaerobic infections	He stops the Abominable Snowball when baseball coach is not available. He doesn't need O_2 to play ball.

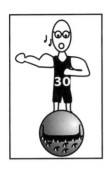

Spectinomycin

mech   30s ribosome
Rt   Single IM injection
Tox   Mild
Uses   Gonorrhea

Wears Spectacles

A young player
Muscular
Young ⇒ fewer problems
He has a gondola to woo the women.
   He is the only basketball player
   concerned with this because he is
   the youngest.

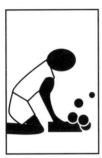

Polymyxin B

mech   Exerts detergent like action and lyses
          bacterial cell membrane
Rt   Parenteral and topical

Tox   Renal
        Neuromuscular like aminoglycosides

Polly the Janitor

Washes floor with soap that dissolves
   court
A parent of players and only works
   after game is over
Goes to showers after the game
Cuts nets down and has same things
   wrong with her as the hockey
   referee

Aminoglycosides—Hockey

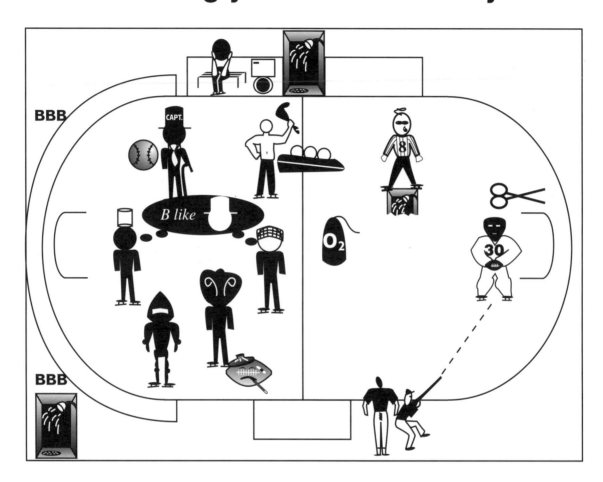

Picture Key

This is a picture of a hockey game in which the aminoglycosides are on offense and their opponents are the bacteria. The idea behind this game is for the hockey player to either make a goal on the bacteria or to knock the bacteria out.

Body	Rink
Aminoglycosides	Hockey players
Skin or before entry to body	Bench
Toxicity	Damage that is inflicted upon referee #8
Kidney	The showers in the locker room
CSF	Bleachers
Blood–Brain Barrier (BBB)	Glass wall protecting spectators
Penicillins	Baseball player
Cephalosporins	Football player
Bacterial cell membrane	The net of the goal
Bacteria	Goal
30s ribosome	Goalie is 30 years old

Aminoglycosides in General

N	All end in -cin; most end in -"mycin"*	They try to <u>sin</u> as much as possible.
	Streptomycin, <u>Gent</u>amicin, <u>K</u>anamycin, <u>A</u>mikacin, <u>T</u>obramycin, <u>N</u>eomycin, <u>N</u>etilmicin	<u>S</u>ome <u>gents</u> <u>k</u>iss <u>a</u>nd <u>t</u>ell <u>n</u>o <u>o</u>ne.
mech	Bacteri<u>cidal</u>[†]	<u>Rough</u> sport
	If O_2 is present, aminoglycosides are actively transported into bacteria	Goalie is out of breath, so if there is O_2 around the goalie will let them score.
	Inhibit 30s ribosome	The goalie is 30 years old and has "30" on his shirt.
	Damages cell <u>membrane</u>	Hockey player use scissors to cut the <u>net</u> of the goal so that they can try to sneak the puck into the goal.
Dist	Can't cross <u>BBB</u>	Hockey player can't get over <u>glass wall</u>.
Met	Almost 100% excreted in <u>urine</u> unchanged	All hockey players go to the <u>showers</u> after the game.
Tox	See toxicities at end of chapter	Referee #8's injuries
Rt	<u>IV</u> and <u>IM</u>	They have <u>ivory</u> hockey sticks and all hockey players are <u>muscular</u>.
Uses	Only <u>aerobic</u> G[–] <u>bacilli</u>	O_2 is required for the goalie to let the player score goals.
		When the goalie is shaped like a <u>football</u>, they really get him.
R_x/R_x	Synergism with β lactamase antibiotics → increased entry into bacteria	Baseball and football players[‡] shoot the goalie, making it easier for the hockey player to score a goal.
Res	Plasmid-mediated c<u>onjugation</u> of aminoglycoside	After goalie gets too many goals scored on him, he gets mad and <u>hits</u> the hockey players with his stick.
	<u>Decreased penetration</u> of aminoglycoside	Goalie learns the hockey players' tricks, and he gets better at defending against them so they <u>can't score</u> as easily.

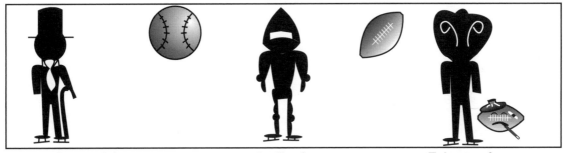

	Gentamicin	**Amikacin**	**Tobramycin**

N	<u>Gent</u>amicin	A <u>gent</u>leman hockey player
	<u>A</u>mikacin	Hockey player who wears extensive <u>armor</u>.
	<u>To</u>bramycin	<u>Cobra</u> hockey player
mech	Amikacin is resistant to plasmid-mediated conjugation	The armor protects amikacin from the goalie's hockey stick.
Uses	Used in infections until sensitivities for the bacteria are determined	The <u>gentle</u>man is sent out to meet the goalie first.
	Broad spectrum	They can beat just about any goalie ⇒ broad coverage.

*Note: Not all antibiotics that end in -mycin are aminoglycosides. Macrolides also end in -mycin.

[†]Note: Cidal, even though they are protein synthesis inhibitors.

[‡]Rem: The penicillins are baseball players, and cephalosporins are football players.

Bacterial endocarditis with a <u>penicillin</u>.

Hospital acquired G⁻ infections
Amikacin can be used for G⁻ infections
   <u>resistant</u> to other aminoglycosides.
<u>Tobra</u>mycin is more active vs. <u>Pseudomonas</u>.

Can get help from <u>baseball players</u> when it is a
   dangerous infection.

The goalie cannot kill amikacin because of his
   armor, even if the goalie has a <u>hockey stick</u>.
The <u>cobra</u> loves to eat <u>hypochondriacs</u> (i.e.,
   pseudo + moaners).

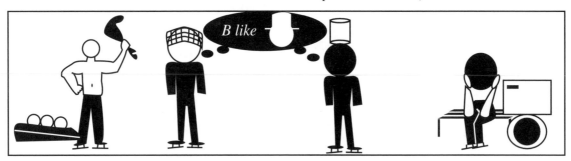

Streptomycin   **Netilmicin**   **Kanamycin**   **Neomycin**

N	<u>Strep</u>tomycin	<u>Stripping</u> hockey player
	<u>Net</u>ilmicin	A hockey player who wears a hair n<u>et</u>
	<u>Kan</u>amycin	Hockey player wearing a <u>can</u> on his head
	<u>Neo</u>mycin	The <u>new</u>* boy, the rookie hockey player
Uses	Resistance has limited the usefulness of streptomycin	Since the stripper is naked → goalie already "knows" all of his tricks. Because of this, it is easier for the goalie to defend against the stripper.
	Streptomycin can be used as a secondary agent for <u>tuberculosis</u>	If the goalie is a <u>bobsledder</u>†, then the goalie will let the stripper make some goals until the <u>bobsledder</u> gets used to the game and begins to play skillfully.
	Netilmicin and kanamycin are similar to gentamicin	These two hockey players want to be like the gent.
	Neomycin—<u>topical</u> applications on wounds and <u>bowel</u> preparation prior to surgery	Since he is a rookie, he remains on the <u>bench</u> and he gets the dirty job of cleaning <u>toilets.</u>

Aminoglycoside Toxicities

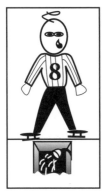

Toxiticities are severe enough to limit duration of treatment and may even prohibit the use of aminoglycosides.

<u>Renal</u> toxicity

8th nerve damage—<u>vestibular</u> and <u>auditory</u>
   by direct toxicity to the hair cells

Hyper<u>sensitivity</u>
<u>Neuromuscular</u> blockade

Referee #8's Injuries

The hockey players throw him into
   the <u>showers.</u>

Referee #8: hockey players spin him
   until he gets <u>dizzy</u> and hit him in
   the ears → go <u>deaf</u>.
They make him <u>cry</u>.
Bodycheck him → <u>paralysis</u> of
   muscles

---

*Neo = new, even though neomycin is not the "new" drug.
†Rem: Bobsledder ⇒ tuberculosis throughout *The Phunny Pharm*.

Quinolones—Wrestling

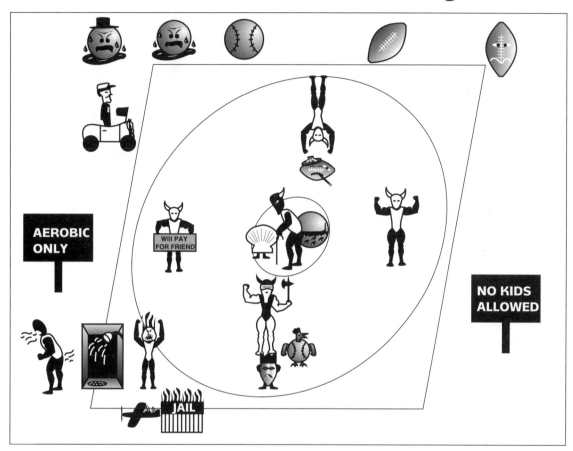

Picture Key

This picture is of the "Oxen" wrestling team—the quinolones. The drugs are represented as players on the team and the mat is the body. The important point with this family is to learn the general points about quinolones well, because all of the drugs in this family are very similar.

Quinolones	Wrestlers
Body	Wrestling mat
Bacteria	Opponents
Toxicities	Things that can happen to the wrestlers

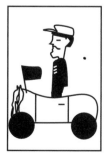

Nalidixic Acid
Uses   Not generally used

The Coach ⇒ <u>Now</u> the <u>Dictator</u>
Since he is the dictator (i.e., the coach), he doesn't get to wrestle.

Quinolones

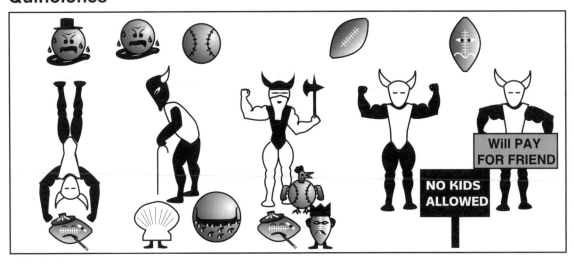

	Ciprofloxacin	Ofloxacin	Norfloxacin	Enoxacin	Lomefloxacin

N	All are relatives of <u>nalidixic</u> acid, but the currently used ones all end in -<u>oxacin</u>:
	   Cipro<u>flox</u>acin
	   O<u>flox</u>acin
	   Nor<u>flox</u>acin
	   <u>Enox</u>acin
	   Lome<u>flox</u>acin
				The <u>dictator</u>
				All are on the -<u>oxen</u> wrestling team
				   Reciprocal <u>oxen</u> ⇒ likes standing on his hands
				   The <u>ol'</u> <u>oxen</u>
				   A big guy, he is a <u>norse oxen</u>
				   <u>Eno</u> the big and bad <u>oxen</u>
				   The <u>lonely</u> <u>oxen</u>		

mech	Inhibit DNA <u>gyrase</u> Bactericidal			Inhibit the <u>gyration</u> of the other wrestlers This is a very rough sport.		
Dist	Well distributed throughout the body					
Tox	GI CNS (dizziness and tremors) Photosensitivity Can't use in prepuberty because of cartilage erosion (FDA-approved only in > 18 years old)			Wrestlers don't eat a lot. Can land on head and get dizzy They wear sunglasses. Because these wrestling matches are so rough, only adults are allowed to watch ⇒ over 18 years old.		
Rt	PO and parenteral					
Uses	**Effective only vs. <u>aerobes</u>** Broad spectrum ⇒ many G⁻ and G⁺ Staphylococcus and methicillin-resistant staph <u>Hemophilis influenzae</u> Effective for <u>Pseudomonas</u> All can be used for UTIs Ciprofloxacin is the most effective vs. <u>Pseudomonas</u> Ofloxacin also used for <u>Neisseria gonorrhoeae</u> and <u>chlamydia</u> Norfloxacin also used for UTIs caused by <u>Enterococcus</u>, <u>Enterobacter</u>, or <u>Pseudomonas</u>			<u>Aerobic</u> sport They are tough and will wrestle just about anyone. Like to wrestle the Abominable Snowball and the MR Wrestle the <u>crazy man</u>. Wrestlers hate <u>hypochondriacs.</u> They can all go to the shower. Reciprocal gets the <u>hypochondriacs</u> the best. There is a <u>gondola</u> and a <u>clam</u> next to the ol' oxen. The norse oxen can tackle the <u>terrible cock,</u> the <u>bad emperor,</u> and the <u>hypochondriac,</u>		
R_x/R_x	Mg^{+2}, Al^{+3} antacids ↓s absorption Cimetidine ↓s renal clearance and ↑s $t_{1/2}$ of quinolones Quinolones ↑ theophylline levels Quinolones ↑ anticoagulant effect of coumadin					

Other Agents for Urinary Tract Infections (UTIs)

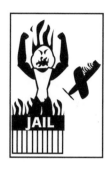

Nitrofurantoin

N   Nitrofurantoin

Tox   N/V
       Pulmonary interstitial fibrosis
       Peripheral neuropathy
       Hepatotoxicity
Rt   PO
Uses Prophylaxis of UTIs

Nitro, Who Is furious

A wrestler named Nitro who can
     become extremely furious
Vomiting
Nitro can also injure the airport.*

Burns the jail
He yells very loud when he is furious.
He looks so mean that he can be used
     just to prevent a confrontation.

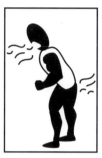

Methenamine

N   Methenamine

mech Breaks down to formaldehyde
       in the acidic environment of
       the urine

Rt   PO
Uses Not for use with urea-splitting
       organisms (e.g., Proteus), because
       methenamine is not broken down
       Prophylaxis for UTIs

Methane

They call him methane because he has
     a lot of flatulence.
He smells so bad, he smells like
     formaldehyde (he is probably a first
     year medical student in anatomy
     lab).
His breath also stinks.
He cannot beat Proteus.

He usually doesn't even have to get
     on the mat in order to win because
     he smells so bad ⇒ he prevents
     confrontations

---

*Rem: The airport represents the lungs, as will be seen in the tuberculosis, asthma, and general anesthesia chapters.

Antituberculosis Chemotherapy—Bobsledding

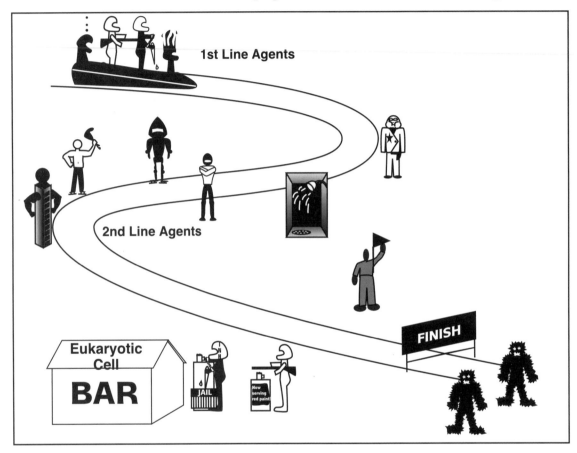

Picture Key

Because tuberculosis mainly affects the lungs, this picture is of a game that is played in the tubes and runways that represent the lung. This representation of the lung will correlate with the pictures that occur in the anesthesia and asthma chapters. It depicts a bobsledding track in which the drugs are attempting to make their way down the course. If they make it to the bottom, then they kill the mycobacterium. The first-line drugs are on the bobsled, and the second-line drugs are around the track and attempt to help the first-line drugs reach the bottom.

Mycobacteria tuberculosis	The bad guys at the finish line at the bottom of the bobsled run
First-line antimycobacterials	The bobsledders already on the "four-man team"
Second-line antimycobacterials	The bobsledders scattered along the track who are trying to help the main sledders get down the track
Mycolic acid an important part of the mycobacterial cell wall	The finish line tape that is strung across the track
Mycobacteria that are within eukaryotic cells	Eukaryotic cells are the bar, and if a drug can penetrate a eukaryotic cell then that drug can enter the bar.

Liver — The policeman of the sledding course
Kidney — The showers
Toxicity — The bobsledding fan at the end of the course

First-Line Antimycobacterials

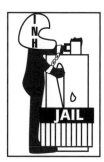

Isoniazid

N	Isoniazid	

The Captain ⇒ "Ice on the Skid"

The captain of the bobsledding team puts Ice on the Skid to allow the sled to run faster so they can hit the bad guys at the end of the run harder.

mech — Inhibits synthesis of mycolic acid (a component of the cell walls) — Ice on the Skid breaks the tape at the finish line.

Dist — Penetrates eukaryotic cells — Goes to the bar after the finish line to finish off the rest of the mycobacteria

Met — N-acetylation by liver — "Hand-cuffed" by the track policeman*

Tox — Can also remember by **INH** — "**INH:** **I**ces **N**erves and **H**epatocytes"

Rate of acetylation correlated with peripheral neuropathy (more common in slow acetylators) — Need to hand-cuff quickly or Ice on the Skid will get frostbitten and will not be able to feel his hands.

Hepatic damage (most common in fast acetylators) — If cop tries to hand-cuff Ice on the Skid too fast then he will get the cop.

Rt — PO — Chews ice

R_x/R_x — Increased incidence of hepatic damage with EtOH — If cop is drunk, then he will really get iced.

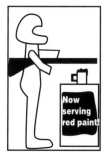

Rifampin

N	Rifampin	

Rifleman

Rifleman shoots the bad guys at the finish.

mech — Inhibits initiation of RNA synthesis by inhibition of RNA polymerase — Shoots the runt puppy factory†

Dist — Penetrates eukaryotic cells — Rifleman goes to the bar after they get to the finish line to finish off the rest of the mycobacteria.

Met — Induces P-450 enzymes — If misses sled then he will hit the fan and the fan will be influenced for the worse‡

Tox — Immunologic reactions → severe flu-like syndrome

Renal and bone marrow toxicity — He shoots the shower and the fan's bones.

Red-colored urine and sweat — He paints the fan red with blood if he shoots him.

Rt — PO — Bites the bullet

Uses — Also used in exposure to meningococci, H. influenzae, and carrier state of MRSA — Also used to eliminate the crazy man and MR. Abominable Snowball

---

*Rem: N-acetylation ⇒ hand-cuffed throughout *The Phunny Pharm* and signifies getting him off of the course.

†Rem: RNA synthesis is represented by the Runt Puppy Factory throughout *The Phunny Pharm*. See upcoming antiviral and antineoplasm chapters.

‡Rem: Influenza virus ⇒ a bad influence steer, as can be seen in the following antiviral chapter.

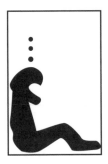

Ethambutol

mech	Inhibits mycolic acid synthesis ⇒ inhibits cell wall synthesis	
Dist	Doesn't penetrate eukaryotic cells but concentrates in lung	
Tox	Optic neuritis—loss of central vision and red-green color blindness	
	Gastrointestinal	

Ethanol Man

Gets the bad guys drunk so that they forget to put up the finish line tape

He is so drunk that they do not allow him in the bar.

Fan may get blind drunk.

Pyrazinamide

Tox	Hepatotoxicity	
	Inhibits uric acid excretion	
Rt	PO	

Pyromaniac in the Sled

He likes to burn the jail.

He yells with joy as he burns things.

Second-Line Antimycobacterials

The definition of what constitutes a second-line antimycobacterial is continually changing. Some believe streptomycin is actually a first-line agent.

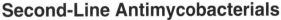

Streptomycin	Amikacin	PAS	Cycloserine

N	Streptomycin (see also aminogycosides)	Hockey player who is a stripper sits on the side of the run and helps the first-line agents down the course.
	Amikacin	Hockey player who wears extensive armor
	p-aminosalicylic acid (PAS)	PEZ candy man
	Cycloserine	The psycho
mech	Streptomycin and amikacin are only effective vs. extracellular TB.	Not allowed in the bar because one is naked and the other wears armor.
	PAS is similar to sulfonamides	The PEZ candy man is a water polo player.
	Cycloserine inhibits cell wall synthesis	The psycho runs around like a crazy man and keeps the mycobacteria from putting up the finish line tape.
Tox	PAS causes GI side effects	The PEZ candy man feeds the fan too much candy and he gets sick.
	Cycloserine → convulsions and psychotic episodes	Causes the fan to go crazy (i.e., psycho)
Uses	Can be used in multi-drug resistant TB and atypical mycobacteria	

Antifungals—Golf

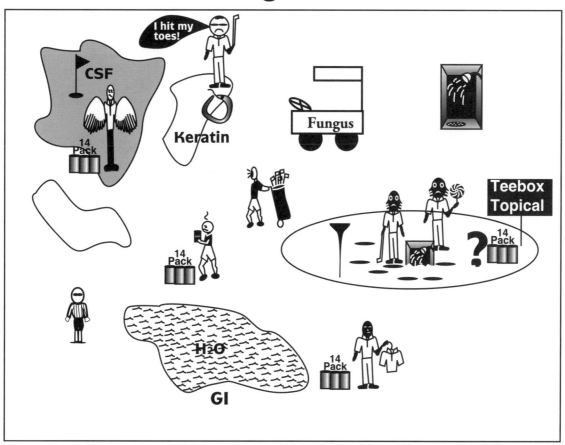

Picture Key

In this picture, the golfers are trying to hit their balls such that they destroy the "fungal golf cart." The body is the golf course, and different areas on the course are areas within the body. An important part of the antifungals involves the ability of the drug to reach the site of infection. Therefore, an essential part of making this picture work involves remembering the location of the drug in the picture and the meaning of the area in which the drug is located.

Body	Golf course
Antifungals	The golfers trying to hit the "fungal golf cart"
Fungi	Golf carts that run around the course, interfere with the golfers' game, and destroy the course
Keratin	Sand trap
CSF	On the green
Topical	In the tee box
Systemic	Not in the tee box
Kidney	The shower on the course
Hepatic	Golf referee
Gastrointestinal tract	H_2O hazard

Polyenes in General

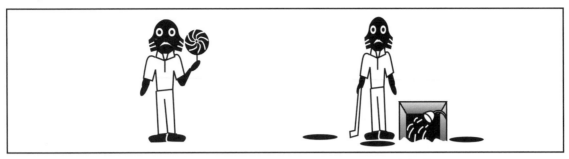

		Nystatin	**Amphotericin B**
N		Nystatin	New starter ⇒ the rookie
		Amphotericin B	Amphibian who terrorizes kids
mech		Bind ergosterol → disruption of membrane integrity	They both put holes in the fungal golf cart by steering their balls to hit the fungal carts.
Dist		Not absorbed from GI tract	They both hit one ball into the H_2O hazard.
Rt		Nystatin ⇒ PO and topical	He is eating candy and standing in the tee box.
		Amphotericin B ⇒ PO for intestinal infections, intrathecal for CSF infections, IV slowly for systemic infections	Can get to the green if he cheats* by throwing it onto the green, and he uses his ivory clubs once he is out on the fairway
Uses		Nystatin ⇒ candidal infections	Still a kid and likes candy, such that if the fungal golf cart is the candy man, he will try put holes in it
		Amphotericin B ⇒ most widely used antifungal Severe fungal infections, but still have to live with the poor therapeutic index	A very good golfer when he uses the ivory but still makes a lot of divots and therefore damages the golf course.
Tox		Azotemia	
		Amphotericin B ⇒ poor therapeutic index Fever and chills	He makes a lot of divots when he plays. He gets hot and cold when out of H_2O too long because he is an amphibian.
		Nephrotoxicity ↓ magnesium and phosphorous	He terrorizes (i.e., breaks) the showers.

Imidazoles in General

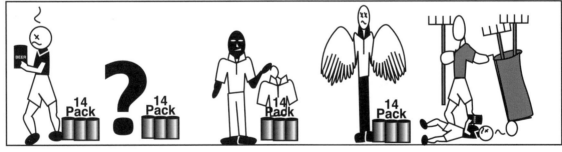

Ketoconazole Miconazole   Clotrimazole   Fluconazole   Itraconazole

N		All end in -azole	A hole
		Ketoconazole	Drinking ketone beer because he made it off of the tee box
		Miconazole	My contraceptive trying to hit the fungal cart
		Clotrimazole	Trying on clothes trying to hit the fungal cart

*Injecting the antifugal intrathecally seems like cheating, but it works clinically.

	Fluconazole	Flew onto green in one shot
	Itraconazole	It golfs with rakes as golf clubs.
mech	Inhibits synthesis of ergosterol (14-α-demethylase)	They all inhibit the steering ability of the fungal golf carts with 14-packs of beer.
Dist	Ketoconazole ⇒ does not enter CSF	Still on the fairway
	Fluconazole ⇒ excellent penetration into CSF	Hit the ball onto the green in one shot
Met	Ketoconazole ⇒ Hepatic	Against the rules to drink on the course; therefore, the golf referee can get him
Tox	Ketoconazole ⇒ inhibits synthesis of steroids	If he drinks too much beer, then he will become sterile.*
	Fluconazole ⇒ allergic rash, GI, Stevens–Johnson syndrome	
Rt	Ketoconazole ⇒ PO	Drinking ketone beer on the fairway
	Miconazole and clotrimazole ⇒ topical	Still in the teebox
	Fluconazole ⇒ PO and IV	Drinking beer and can use his ivory clubs
Uses	Ketoconazole ⇒ systemic fungal infections	Hits ball onto the green
	Histoplasmosis	Especially likes to get the golf cart drunk if it
	Coccidioidomycosis	has snakes (i.e., "Hssss") or roosters (i.e., cocks) driving
	Blastomycosis	Likes to blast the golf carts
	Miconazole ⇒ vaginal candidiasis	(Not touching this one either)
	Fluconazole ⇒ cryptococcus	He attacks the golf cart from the crypt.
	Candida (oral and esophageal)	Rewards himself with some candy from the candyman golf cart
	Coccidioidomycosis	Especially likes to hit the golf cart if there are roosters (i.e., cocks) driving it
	Itraconazole ⇒ may replace ketoconazole in treatment of Aspergillus	It rakes ketoconazole up when he is too drunk to stand.
R_x/R_x	Ketoconazole and itraconazole have ↓ absorption with R_x that ↓ gastric acidity. Also inhibit P450	Ketoconazole and itraconazole do not play well if there is no acid around.

Others

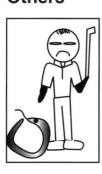

	Griseofulvin	**The Greasy Golfer**
mech	Deposits in keratin-containing tissues	On his second shot, from the H_2O, he landed in the sand trap, so he's mad.
	Uptake energy-dependent	Takes energy to get out of sand trap
	Inhibits mitosis	He says, "I hit my toes."
Tox	GI	Gets sick after he drinks H_2O from H_2O hazard
	Headache and coma	It's a headache to get out of the pit.
Rt	PO administration with fatty meals	Eats greasy meals
Uses	Tinea (i.e., ringworm)	The ringworm lives in the sand pit
	Dermatophytes of hair, skin, and nails	and greasy golfer kills him with his club.

*Rem: Testosterone is needed for fertility.

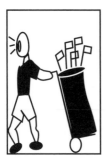

Flucytosine

N   Flu<u>cy</u>tosine

mech   Inhibits DNA synthesis

Uses   Not used alone because resistance
        develops rapidly

The Caddie with Great <u>Sight</u>

The caddie with great <u>sight</u> needs the
good sight to help the golfers in
their games.
The caddie can hit the dogs in
alignment* of the fungi.
He is a caddie; he only helps the
golfers but will not play alone.

Potassium Iodide (i.e., KI)

Rt   Topical   Remains in the <u>tee box</u>
Uses   Sporotrichosis

---

*Rem: DNA synthesis is dogs in alignment throughout *The Phunny Pharm*. See the upcoming antiviral and antineoplasm chapters.

Antimalarial Chemotherapy—Pool

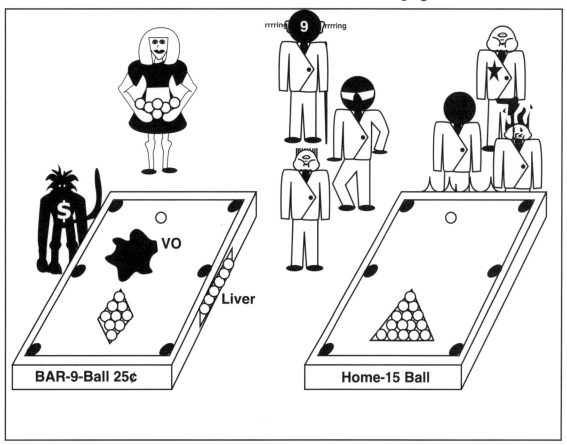

Plasmodia Summary

Malaria is caused by the Plasmodia family, but as with any family, there are numerous species within it. *Plasmodia falciparum* and *P. malariae* are the two species that only infect red blood cells without infecting the liver. In contrast, *P. vivax* and *P. ovale* infect hepatocytes as well as red blood cells. As a result, if only red blood cells are treated, the hepatocytes can be a source of relapse. Therefore, in order to produce a complete cure with these last two species, the tissue phase must also be treated.

Picture Key

In this picture, the game is pool, wherein the antimalarial drugs are the pool players and malaria is the pool balls on the table. The object of the game is for the pool players to clear the table of the malarial balls.

Two types of infection (i.e., blood and liver [tissue])	Two types of pool tables (i.e., home and bar tables)
In the blood	On the table
Plasmodia	Pool balls
Antimalarials	Pool players
To kill plasmodia	To knock balls into pockets
Red blood cell	Rack for balls
Severe infections (i.e., more bugs in the blood)	More balls on the table

<u>Mosquito</u> injects plasmodia into body	<u>Waitress</u> (not quite a "bar fly") puts more balls on table
Parasitized RBC	Balls racked and ready to be broken
All can be administered <u>PO</u>	<u>PO</u>ol

Plasmodium Species Review

Plasmodium Species
With a Tissue Phase

P.<u>v</u>ivax and *P.<u>o</u>vale*

<u>Liver</u>

Some plasmodia remain in liver and therefore can be a source for relapse
To kill tissue plasmodia

To attack erythrocyte phase
To attack tissue (i.e., liver) phase

Without a Tissue Phase

P. falciparum and <u>P.</u> *malariae*
No tissue phase

All plasmodia are in the blood

In the Phunny Pharm
The Bar Pool Table

<u>V.O.</u> ⇒ vodka is spilt on the table at the bar
The <u>ball chamber</u> (fittingly, the bar table has a liver to digest the EtOH that is spilt upon it)
Only play 9-ball at the bar (i.e., 6 balls always remain in the ball chamber)
Need money to remove balls from the ball chamber as well as be able to play pool
Play pool and knock balls in the holes
Use money to remove balls from the ball chamber.

The Home Pool Table

There is no ball chamber in this table—the balls land in "nets" in each pocket ⇒ money is not needed to play.
Play 8-ball (in 8-ball you use all 15 balls)

Antimalarials

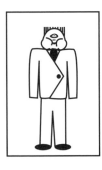

Chloroquine

N	<u>Chloroquine</u>
mech	Parasitized RBCs concentrate R_x
Tox	Retinal degeneration (after years of use)
	Hemolysis in G6PD–deficient patients
Uses	Acute attacks ($\underline{R}_x$ of choice)
	Only acts on erythrocytic stage

A <u>Cyclops</u> Who Likes to <u>Win</u>

A <u>cyclops</u>, named <u>Chlor</u>, who likes to <u>win</u> at pool
Loves to break when balls are racked
Lost one eye when he played too long

<u>Best</u> <u>player</u> when lots of balls on table
Only plays the game but cannot afford to get more balls out of the chamber when he is through

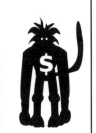

Primaquine

mech	Kills tissue forms only
Tox	Hemolytic anemia in G6PD deficiency
Uses	Kills tissue forms only; therefore, always used in combination with other R_xs

A <u>Primate</u> Who Likes to <u>Win</u>— He Is the Manager

He has money to support his players and take the balls out of the chamber, but he can't play pool because he is too short.

Primate supplies money, but he needs the other players to play for him in order to win.

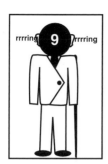

Quinine

mech	Parasitized RBCs concentrate R$_x$	
	Interferes with <u>metabolism</u> (DNA)	
Tox	<u>Cinch</u>onism (temporary)	
		Ears—tinnitus and deafness
		Eyes—decreased acuity, field of vision, and blind
		Headache
Rt	Also <u>IV</u> for life threatening	
Uses	Only acts on erythrocytic stage	
	When resistant to <u>chloroquine</u>	

Wins at 9-ball

Loves to break when balls are racked
Hits balls so hard that they can't <u>eat</u>
When he plays too much, he thinks
    game is a <u>cinch</u>.
    Loud music in bar → ears start to
        ring and he goes deaf
    Because a cinch, he tries to play
        drunk → blurry vision. He drinks
        so much he goes blind and gets a
        headache.
Will use his <u>ivory</u> cue when he has a
    lot of balls on table and is in a
    serious game
Only plays pool; he has no money to
    get the balls out of the chamber
He will play if <u>cyclops</u> can't win.

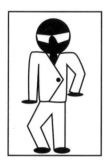

Mefloquine

Uses	Only for chloroquine resistance	
	Prophylaxis of infection	

The <u>Mellow Winner</u>

If cyclops can't win, the mellow
    winner will take over the game.
He is so mellow that he can be used
    to prevent games.

Tetrahydrofolate Synthesis Inhibitors in General

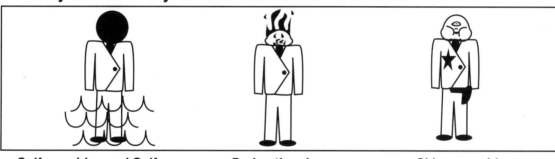

	Sulfonamides and Sulfones	**Pyrimethamine**	**Chloroguanide**
N	Sulfonamides and Sulfones		The water polo players who play pool
	<u>Pyri</u>methamine		A <u>pyro</u>maniac who plays pool
	<u>Chlor</u>o<u>guan</u>ide		A <u>cyclops</u> who <u>guar</u>ds pool games
mech	Inhibit dihydrofolate reductase or dihydropteroate synthase		
Tox	Bone marrow suppression		Dries up bones
	Chloroguanide is the least toxic antimalarial.		Because he is a guard, he does not hurt anyone.
Uses	Acts at erythrocyte, gametocyte, and tissue stage		They have a little money, can play pool, and keep waitress from putting more balls on the table.
	Only in prophylaxis, suppressive treatment, and chloroquine resistance		They are not very good, so they are used if "cyclops who likes to win" can't win.
	Only used with synergistic R$_x$		Water polo player, pyromaniac, and the cyclops guard play doubles ⇒ they are not good enough to play alone.

Antiparasitics—Bowling

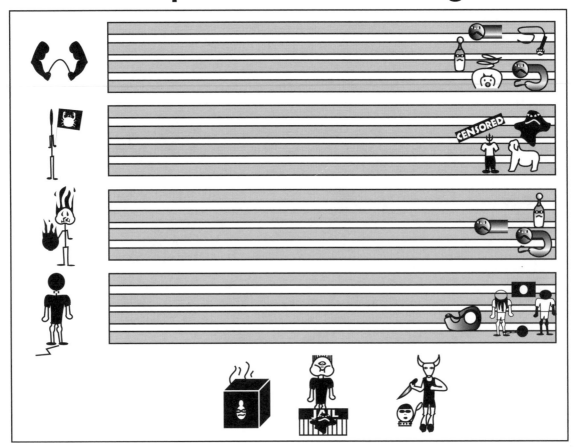

Picture Key

This is a picture of a bowling alley, in which the antiparasitics are the bowlers and the parasites are the balls and pins and other things on the lane that will be bowled down. The object is for the bowlers to knock out the parasites.

GI tract	The bowling lane
Body	The whole bowling alley
Antiparasites	Bowlers
Antiparasites that paralyze	If name begins with "P," then its mechanism is paralyzing the bug → parasite to migrate through the GI tract with the feces, until it is expelled
Central nervous system	The study room in the bowling alley*
Liver	The referee of the bowling game

*Rem: The central nervous system is represented by the University throughout *The Phunny Pharm*. Here it is simply the study room.

Introduction to Parasites

Protozoa

Entamoeba histolytica

Assoc/   Cyst is ingested and then can go
Life   one of four routes:
       1. The patient can pass cysts
          asymptomatically.
       2. <u>Mild</u> GI disease
       3. <u>Severe</u> GI disease
       4. Hepatic <u>abscess</u>
T_x Metronidazole

Amoeba on the Lane

Giardia lamblia

Assoc/   1. Cyst is ingested
Life   2. Becomes a <u>tropho</u>zoite
       3. Cysts bud off and are shed in feces.
T_x Metronidazole

Guardian of the **Lambs**—
    Sheepdog

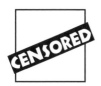

Trichomonas vaginalis

Assoc/   Remains in female vagina or male
Life   urethra
T_x Metronidazole

Vaginal Trick

Cryptosporidium

Assoc/   Infects intestinal epithelial cells
Life
T_x None yet

A Crypt Behind the Lane

It is behind the lane and therefore
   cannot be hit by the bowlers.

Toxoplasma gondii

Assoc/   Cysts from undercooked meat or cat
Life   feces that can get into the brain
T_x Sulfadiazine and pyrimethamine

Toxic Can of Plasma

Leishmaniasis

Assoc/   A flagellate that infects by the bite of
Life   an insect; infects the skin and/or
       viscera
T_x Sodium stibogluconate

Leashman Who Is Mean

Helminths

Ascaris lumbricoides

Assoc/   *Ascaris* ⇒ the round worms that live
Life   in human large intestines. They can
       grow to amazing lengths. Larvae
       travel to the lung.

T_x Mebendazole
        Pyrantel

Scary Balls

Ascaris can get large enough to <u>scare</u>
   the H___ out of you if they crawl
   out your nose. They are the scary
   balls (i.e., round) at the end of
   the lane.

Necator americanus

Assoc/   *Necator americanus* ⇒ the <u>hook</u>worm
Life   similar to *Ascaris* but enter through
       the skin on the feet
T$_x$ Mebendazole

Hook Balls

The <u>hook</u> on the ball at the end of the
lane

Enterobius vermicularis

Assoc/   *Enterobius vermicularis* ⇒ the
Life   <u>pin</u>worms that live in the ileum,
       cecum, and colon. The adult worms
       migrate out the anus and deposit
       eggs in the perianal region. The eggs
       hatch and return to the large intestine
       or go to someone else to live.
T$_x$ Mebendazole
       Pyrantel

Bowling Pins

The bowling <u>pin</u>s at the end of the
lane

Trichuris trichiura

Assoc/   *Trichuris trichiura* ⇒ the whipworms
Life   that remain in the cecum and produce
       eggs that exit in feces
T$_x$ Mebendazole

<u>Tricky</u> <u>Whips</u> in the Lane

The <u>tricky</u> <u>whips</u> in the lane

Trichinella spiralis

Assoc/   *Trichinella spiralis* ⇒ ingestion of
Life   larvae in cysts present in raw
       pork → larvae mature to adults
       and mate → the females produce
       larvae that migrate to organs and
       skeletal muscle
T$_x$ Mebendazole

Tricky Pig with Spiral Tail

The tricky pig with spiral tail in the
lane. These tricky pigs are all over
the bowling alley.

Trematodes (Flukes)

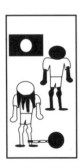

Schistosoma

Assoc/   *Schistosoma* ⇒ a blood fluke.
Life   Eggs are ingested, and adults
       migrate to venules throughout
       the body, where they live (e.g.,
       S. mansoni and S. japonicum live
       in venules of the intestine).
T$_x$ Praziquantel

Manson and Japanese Flukes

Cestodes (Tapeworms)

Taenia

Assoc/   *Taenia solium* ⇒ pork tapeworm that
Life   can form cysts in brain and skeletal
       muscles
       Taenia saginata ⇒ beef tapeworm that
       remains in the intestine
T$_x$ Praziquantel

<u>Tape</u>worms in the Lane

Antiprotozoals

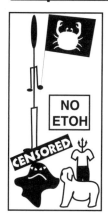

Metronidazole

Dist	Crosses BBB	
	Systemic absorption	
Met	Hepatic	
Tox	Carcinogenic	
	Disulfiram-like reaction	
Rt	PO or IV	
Uses	Broad spectrum:	
	All amebiasis except asymptomatic cyst	
	Hepatic abscess	
	Any anaerobic bacterial infection originating from below the diaphragm	
	Giardia lamblia	
	Entamoeba histolytica	
	Trichomonas vaginalis	
	Clostridium difficile taken PO	

Metra Is as Skinny as a Pole

She can go into the study room.
She can move all over the bowling alley.
If she gets mad at the referee, he will throw her out of game.
Her sign is Cancer—the crab.
Won't allow EtOH on the team, because she knows that it will make them sick
Yells at team, and she uses ivory to keep her skin soft

Only attacks the things in the alley that are causing problems
Can get the enemies that are attacking the bowling referee
She is tough and doesn't need O_2 to play.

She likes to hit the sheepdog.
She likes to hit the amoeba on the lane.
She likes to hit the vaginal trick.
She likes to hit the clothes on a difficult trident.

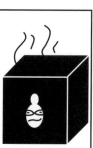

Sodium Stibogluconate

mech	A pentavalent antimony compound that interferes with the protozoal ability to make ATP and GTP	
Uses	*Leishmania*	

A Steer Stabber

He stabs the leash man

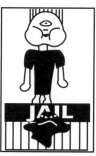

Chloroquine

N	Chloroquine	
Uses	Hepatic amebiasis if metronidazole cannot be used	

Cyclops Pool Player Who Bowls

The cyclops pool player who also likes to win in bowling
Only good at hitting those amoebas that are attacking the bowling referee

Diloxanide Furoate

mech	Amebicidal by an unknown mech	
Met	Remains in GI tract	
Tox	Excessive flatulence	
Rt	PO	
Uses	Asymptomatic cyst carriers	

Locked Inside a Box for What She Ate

Her odor kills cysts.
Is not allowed away from the bowling lane
Locked inside to minimize the odor
Likes to eat a lot
Only allowed to hit opponents that aren't causing a lot of trouble because she is not very good. She can't see them from inside the box.

Antihelmintics

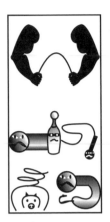

Mebendazole

N	Mebendazole
mech	Disrupts cytoplasmic microtubules
Tox	Teratogenic
Uses	*Ascaris lumbricoides*
	Necator americanus = hookworm
	Enterobius vermicularis = pinworm
	Trichuris trichiura = whipworm
	Trichinella spiralis

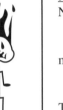

"Me Bend It All"

"Me bend it all"—a big guy who is strong

Throws his bowling ball so hard that he bends the parasites' microtubles

Have to be careful because he does not know his own strength and may "bend babies"

He bends the scary balls.
He bends the hook balls.
He bends the pin.
He bends the whip.
He bends the tricky pig with the spiral tail.

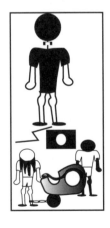

Pyrantel

N	Pyrantel
mech	Paralyzes by depolarizing
Tox	Headache and GI
Rt	Single dose
Uses	*Ascaris lumbricoides*
	Necator americanus = hookworm
	Enterobius vermicularis = pinworm

Pyromaniac Telling of His Deeds

The pyromaniac who lights his ball on fire before he throws it. He tells of his deeds.

Pyrantel turns the pins upside down ⇒ depolarizes them; name begins with a "P" ⇒ paralyzes.

His head is on fire, and he may catch the bowling lane on fire.

Only takes his first throw to finish the job

He hits the scary balls with his burning ball.

He hits the hook ball with his burning ball.

He hits the pin with his burning ball.

Praziquantel

mech	Tetonic contractions → vacuole formation dislodging the parasite
	Paralyzes
	Inhibits egg production
Tox	Low toxicity
Rt	PO
Uses	Cestodes and Trematodes
	Schistosoma
	Taenia

A Bowler Who Prays for a Quake

Quake ≈ tectonic shifts → the schistosomes to lose their footing on the court so that they fall off

Praziquantel begins with a "P" ⇒ paralyzes

This player does not approve of extramarital egg production.

Mild-mannered player

He makes Manson and the Japanese lose their footing.

He makes the tapeworms lose their footing.

Antivirals and Antineoplastics—Dog Racing

Although this is not the Alaskan Iditerod, often it is a race for a patient's life. In viral infections, the cell is misdirected by the virus to produce viral proteins, and neoplastic cells ignore signals that tell normal cells to stop dividing. As a result, the malignant cell proliferates and causes problems. The accessible targets for treatment of viruses and neoplasms are more subtle than those of bacterial infections because the affected cells were once normal. The main target is the machinery used for the synthesis of DNA, RNA, and ultimately proteins.

The picture in this introduction represents the normal cell. Thereafter, adjustments to the picture are made such that the virus or neoplasm is represented.

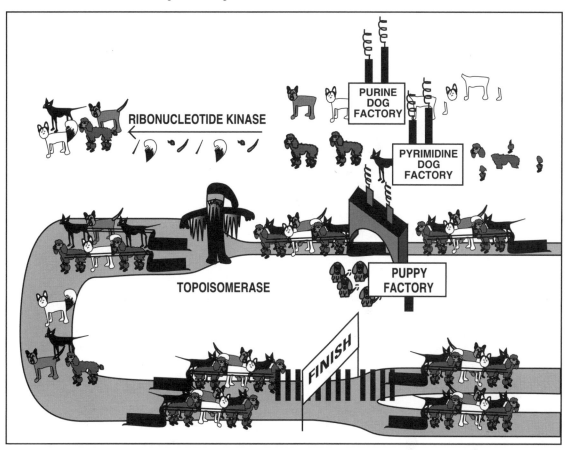

DNA and RNA Primer for the Phunny Pharm: Picture Key for the Normal Cell

This picture depicts the life of a normal cell, the "normal" dog race. This normal life of a cell requires RNA synthesis, which is used for the production of proteins and ultimately the normal function of the cell. When the time is right, the cell prepares itself to divide (i.e., mitosis). In order to do this, the DNA needs to be duplicated. The race is organized such that it depicts all of these parts of the cell's life.

Cell

Purine bases:

   Guanine

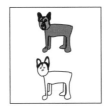

   Adenine

Pyrimidine bases both have a <u>y</u> in their name. They also have one ring in their structure that makes them look like a pie ⇒ one circle.

   <u>Cy</u>tosine

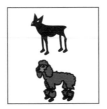

   <u>Thy</u>mine

<u>Nucleosides</u> are purine or pyrimidine bases attached to a <u>sugar</u>

<u>Ribonucleotide kinase</u> responsible for phosphorylation of the nucleoside

<u>Nucleotides</u> are phosphorylated nucleosides that are building blocks for DNA ⇒ nucleosides with a <u>tail</u>

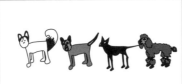

<u>DNA</u>

DNA synthesis:

   <u>G</u>uanine pairs with <u>cy</u>tosine

   <u>A</u>denine pairs with <u>thy</u>mine

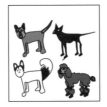

DNA replication ⇒ this must occur before the cell can divide. It ensures that both cells have identical copies of the DNA.

<u>R</u>NA

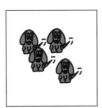

<u>R</u>NA is used to make proteins for the cell

<u>Topoisomerase</u> ⇒ unwinds the DNA for RNA synthesis or DNA replication

<u>The area in which the dog races take place</u>

<u>Pure</u>bred dogs for pulling the sled:

   <u>G</u>erman Shepherds

   Alaskan Malamutes

They have "y" in their names.

<u>Coy</u>ote

<u>Toy</u> Poodle

¢

The <u>owner</u> who places a tail on the dog

     The dogs that have a <u>tail</u>

Dogs <u>in a</u>lignment attached to the sled

Dogs are attached to the sled:

   German Shepherds are placed next to <u>coy</u>otes.

   Alaskan Malamutes are placed next to <u>Toy</u> Poodles.

Before the finish line, the dog team is split into two parts and each member of the two dog teams gets a new partner. When this is finished, there are two identical dog teams and sled.

<u>R</u>unts ⇒ puppies that are copied from the racing dogs at puppy factory

<u>R</u>unts make things for the race.

The <u>top ice man</u> of the <u>race</u> separates the two lines of race dogs so runts can be copied from them and so they can be separated into two dog teams.

Picture Key for the Diseased Cell

If the cell is infected by a virus, it is driven to produce virus. If the cell becomes malignant, it gets out of control, becomes immortal, and reproduces itself faster than normal cells.

Cells	The area in which the dog races take place
Viruses	Bad guys who take over the sled and run the dogs wherever and however fast they want
Cancer	Other bad guys who take over the sled
DNA bases	Dogs used for the races
<u>Antivirals</u>	The things used to slow the dogs down
<u>Antineoplastics</u>	The things used to slow the dogs down

Antivirals—Dog Races and Viral Monsters

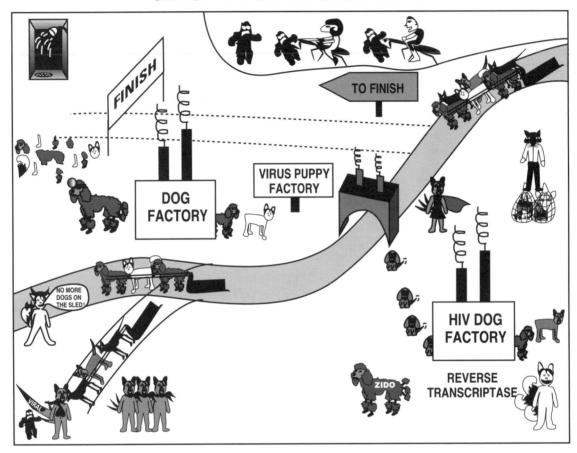

Picture Key

In this section, <u>Phunny Pharm dog races</u> still represent the normal cells. Viruses have infected the cell and the cell is forced to produce viral particles. In the picture, the dogs are distracted from the race by the viral monsters. This not only prevents the dogs from getting to the finish line, but also forces them to make more viral monsters. The antiviral medications are things that interfere with the production of new viral monsters.

Cell	The race course area
Virus	Viral monsters
Entry of the virus into the cell	The viral monster enters the race course area.
Viral reproduction	The viral monster forces the dogs to veer from their normal race course → they are then enslaved to make more viral monsters.
Antivirals	The things that interfere with the production of more viral monsters
<u>Kinases phosphorylate</u> nucleosides to nucleotides before they are incorporated into DNA or RNA.	The <u>owner</u> places a tail on the dogs before they are put on the sled.

Antivirals must be <u>phosphorylated</u> before they can work.

<u>Reverse transcriptase</u> ⇒ an enzyme that synthesizes <u>DNA</u> from viral <u>RNA</u> ("reverse" from usual)
<u>Toxicity</u>

The <u>dog owner</u> places a <u>tail</u> on some of the things that interfere with the production of viral monsters.
An <u>HIV dog factory</u> that copies <u>dogs</u> from the <u>runts</u>

Things that can happen to the person in the sled

Antivirals in General

N	DNA analogs:		Dog impersonators:

N — DNA analogs:
  Guanine analog
    <u>Ribavirin</u>
    <u>Acyclovir</u>
    <u>Ganciclovir</u>
  Adenosine analogs
    <u>Vidarabine</u> (adenine arabinoside, ARA-A)
    Dideoxy<u>inosine</u> (ddI)
  Thymidine analogs
    Ido<u>x</u>uridine
    <u>Zido</u>vudine (<u>AZT</u>)

Dog impersonators:
  German Shepherd impersonators:
    <u>Reb</u>a the <u>villain</u> German Shepherd impersonator
    <u>Ace</u> the <u>clever</u> German Shepherd impersonator
    <u>Gang</u> of <u>clever</u> German Shepherd impersonators
  Alaskan Malamute impersonators:
    <u>Vi</u>king Alaskan Malamute impersonator who is a <u>daring being</u>
    The <u>innocent</u> Alaskan Malamute impersonator
  Toy Poodle impersonators
    <u>Eye doc</u>tor Toy Poodle impersonator
    <u>Zido</u> (like "Fido") the <u>Aztec</u> Toy Poodle impersonator

Inhibitors of viral entry:
  <u>Amantadine</u>
  <u>Rimantadine</u>
Inhibitor of RNA and DNA polymerase:
  <u>Foscarnet</u>

A <u>man</u> riding a <u>mantis</u> that <u>dines</u> on viral monsters
A <u>ram</u> riding a <u>mantis</u> that <u>dines</u> on viral monsters

A <u>fox</u> who uses a <u>net</u>

mech — All DNA analogs are phosphorylated.

All of the viral monster stoppers that look like the dogs need a tail to work.

Met — Almost all are metabolized mainly by the <u>kidney</u>.

All of the viral monster stoppers go to the shower when they are done.

$t_{1/2}$ — All have a longer duration of action than their respective $t_{1/2}$ because their actions depend more upon intracellular availability than blood levels.

¢

Tox — All cause some degree of teratogenicity.

¢: Because drugs interfere with DNA, they will affect the developing fetus.

Uses — <u>The uses are difficult to incorporate into the picture, but are not difficult to memorize:</u>
Ribavirin ⇒ aerosol for respiratory syncytial virus (RSV) in children
Acyclovir ⇒ all herpes simplex infections
  Severe genital infections
  Best R_x for herpes encephalitis
  Zoster = chickenpox
Ganciclovir ⇒ excellent activity vs. CMV
Vidarabine ⇒ type I herpes infection of cornea herpes simplex virus and varicella
Dideoxyinosine ⇒ HIV in zidovudine resistance

Idoxuridine ⇒ type I herpes infection of
  cornea
Zidovudine ⇒ HIV
Amantadine and rimantadine ⇒
  prophylactic to prevent influenza spread;
  shortens duration of influenza symptoms
Foscarnet ⇒ CMV, especially
  CMV-resistant to ganciclovir

Purine Analogs

Guanine Analogs   ## German Shepherd Impersonators

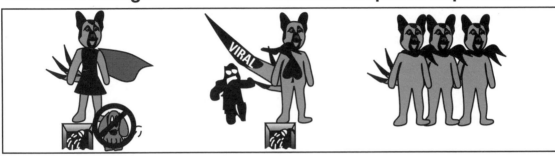

		Ribavirin	**Acyclovir**	**Ganciclovir**

N		Spell <u>RAG</u>:
		  Ribavirin
				There is a <u>RAG</u> around their necks:
				  <u>Reb</u>a the <u>villain</u> German Shepherd
				    impersonator

		Acyclovir Ganciclovir		<u>Ace</u> the <u>clever</u> German Shepherd impersonator <u>Gang</u> of <u>clever</u> German Shepherd impersonators
mech		<u>Guanine</u> <u>analogs</u> are <u>triphosphorylated</u>:		All three German Shepherd impersonators have three tails.

		<u>Ribavirin</u> ⇒ inhibits synthesis of guanine
		  nucleotides and inhibits viral <u>RNA</u>
		  polymerase.
				<u>Reba the villain</u> keeps real German Shepherds
				  from getting their tails and she stops the viral
				  monster's puppy factory. Also note that Reba
				  starts with an "R" and RNA starts with an "R."

		<u>Acyclovir</u> ⇒ <u>different and important</u>:
		  Phosphorylated only in virus-infected
		  cells by **<u>viral</u>** <u>thymidine kinase</u>; 2nd and
		  3rd phosphorylation by the host.
		  Triphosphate stops synthesis of DNA.
				<u>Ace</u> is special:
				  Ace gets his first tail from the viral monster; the
				    second and third, he gets from the usual dog
				    owner.
				  Ace keeps <u>d</u>ogs from being placed <u>in</u>
				    alignment in front of the sled.

		<u>Ganciclovir</u> ⇒ incorporated into DNA →
		  slowing of <u>DNA</u> replication.
				The <u>gang</u> stops <u>d</u>ogs from being placed <u>in</u>
				  alignment in front of the sled.

Tox		Acyclovir ⇒ minimal because it is only
		  active in virus-infected cells.
		  <u>Nephro</u>toxic from crystal formation
		  Less teratogenicity than other antivirals
		    but still must be careful
				<u>Ace</u> only gets its tails after the viral monster gives
				  it the first tail.
				  Ace may damage the <u>showers</u>
				  ¢: Because acyclovir is activated only in cells
				    with virus, the fetus has less problems with it.

		Ganciclovir ⇒ bone marrow suppression → neutropenia		An important clinical fact
Rt		Ribavirin can be by <u>aerosol</u> Ganciclovir ⇒ IV only		Reba the villain uses her cape to <u>fly</u>.
Uses		Ribavirin ⇒ aerosol for respiratory syncytial virus (RSV) in children		

Acyclovir ⇒ all herpes simplex infections
   Severe genital infections
   Best R$_x$ for herpes encephalitis
   Zoster = chickenpox
Ganciclovir ⇒ excellent activity vs. CMV

Adenosine Analogs   ## Alaskan Malamute Impersonators

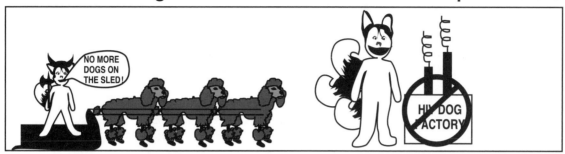

Vidarabine   **Dideoxyinosine**

N	<u>Adenosine Analogs:</u>
	   <u>Vidarabine</u> (adenine arabinoside = ARA-A)
	
	   Dideoxy<u>inosine</u> (ddI)
		<u>A</u>laskan Malamute impersonators:
		   <u>Vi</u>king Alaskan Malamute impersonator who
		      is a <u>daring being</u>
		   The <u>innocent</u> Alaskan malamute impersonator

mech	Both are <u>adenosine analogs</u> that are
	   <u>triphosphorylated</u> and inhibit <u>DNA</u>
	   <u>transcription</u>
	<u>Vidarabine</u> → potent inhibition of <u>DNA</u>
	   polymerase
	Dideoxy<u>inosine</u> → inhibition of <u>reverse</u>
	   <u>transcriptase</u> and <u>DNA</u> synthesis
		They both are <u>Alaskan malamute impersonators</u>
		   that get <u>three tails</u> and stop <u>D</u>ogs from being
		   placed <u>in</u> alignment in front of the sled.
		<u>Viking daring being</u> stops the production of two
		   dog teams from the one.
		The <u>innocent</u> Alaskan Malamute impersonator
		   enters the <u>HIV dog factory</u> and stops it from
		   copying <u>dogs</u> from the HIV monster's <u>runts</u>.

Tox	<u>Vidarabine</u> ⇒ <u>nausea, vomiting, diarrhea</u>
	
	Dideoxy<u>inosine</u> ⇒ peripheral <u>neuropathy,</u>
	   <u>pancreatitis</u>
		The person in the sled gets <u>sick</u> to his stomach
		   when he sees the Viking.
		The <u>innocent</u> Alaskan Malamute makes the
		   person in the sled have <u>pancreas</u> problems.

Rt	<u>Vidarabine</u> ⇒ eyedrops, IV Dideoxy<u>inosine</u> ⇒ <u>PO</u> with antacids	The <u>Viking</u> has big eyes. The <u>innocent</u> has a <u>big mouth</u>.

Uses	<u>Vidarabine</u> type I herpes infection of <u>cornea,</u>
	   herpes symplex virus, and <u>Varicella</u>
	Dideoxy<u>inosine</u> ⇒ HIV in zidovudine
	   resistance
		The <u>innocent</u> gets the HIV monster if Zido, the
		   Aztec Toy Poodle, can't get it.

Pyrimidine Analogs

Thymidine Analogs   ## Toy Poodle Impersonators

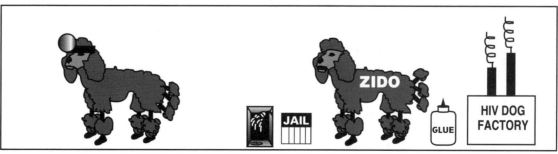

Idoxuridine   **Zidovudine**

N	Idoxuridine	Eye doctor Toy Poodle impersonator
	Zidovudine (AZT)	Zido (like "Fido") the Aztec Toy Poodle impersonator
mech	Thymidine analogs that are triphosphorylated and block DNA replication	They each have three tails and stop dogs from being placed in alignment in front of the sled.
	Idoxuridine ⇒ blocks production of DNA precursors	The eye doctor Toy Poodle impersonator stops the dog factory.
	Zidovudine ⇒ inhibits viral reverse transcriptase → terminating synthesis of DNA from viral RNA	The Aztec Zido is a toy poodle that goes into HIV dog factory and stops it from copying dogs from the HIV monster's runts (puppies).
Met	Zidovudine ⇒ renal and hepatic by glucuronidation	Aztec Zido is sent to the shower and can be glued into jail.*
Tox	Idoxuridine ⇒ selective toxicity is low as eyedrops' systemic absorption is small	
	Zidovudine ⇒ headache, myopathy, bone marrow suppression, severe anemia	The person in the sled has a headache, sore muscles, a broken leg, and is bleeding
Rt	Idoxuridine ⇒ eyedrops	Eye doctor
	Zidovudine ⇒ PO only	Aztec Zido has a large mouth.
Uses	Idoxuridine ⇒ type I herpes infection of cornea	Eye doctor is used to treat eye infections.
	Zidovudine ⇒ HIV	Aztec Zido stops the HIV monster.
R_x/R_x	Zidovudine ⇒ liver toxicity is increased if glucuronidation in liver is decreased by other drugs ⇒ probenecid, acetaminophen, lorazepam, indomethacin, cimetidine. Bone marrow toxicity is increased by ganciclovir.	

Other Antivirals

Inhibitors of Viral Entry

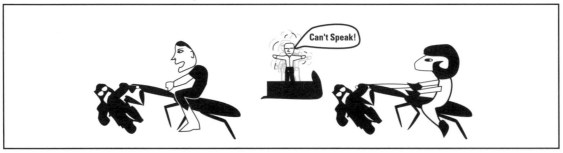

	Amantadine	**Rimantadine**
N	Amantadine	A man riding a mantis that dines on viral monsters
	Rimantadine	A ram riding a mantis that dines on viral monsters
mech	Block penetration and/or uncoating of the virus as it enters the cell	Mantis dines on the viral monsters as they enter the area of the dog races.
Tox	CNS ⇒ irritability, tremor, slurred speech	The man on the sled trembles and can't speak for fear of the mantis.
Rt	PO	Mantis is eating a viral monster.
Uses	Prophylactic to prevent influenza spread; shortens duration of influenza symptoms	

*Rem: Liver is represented by the Phunny Pharm Jail.

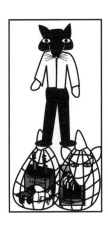

Foscarnet

N   Foscarnet

mech   Inhibits RNA and DNA polymerase

Tox   Renal dysfunction

Electrolyte abnormalities ⇒ binds
   cations—especially decreases
   Ca^{+2} with increasing dose

Rt   IV with large volumes of fluid only

Uses   CMV
           CMV resistant to ganciclovir

Fox Using a Net

A fox who uses a net to entangle the
   virus monster

He nets the puppy factory and stops
   dogs from being placed in
   alignment in front of the sled.

The fox entangles the shower with
   his net.

The fox also nets cows with his net
   and decreases the number of them
   in the body.

Cancer Chemotherapy—Dog Races

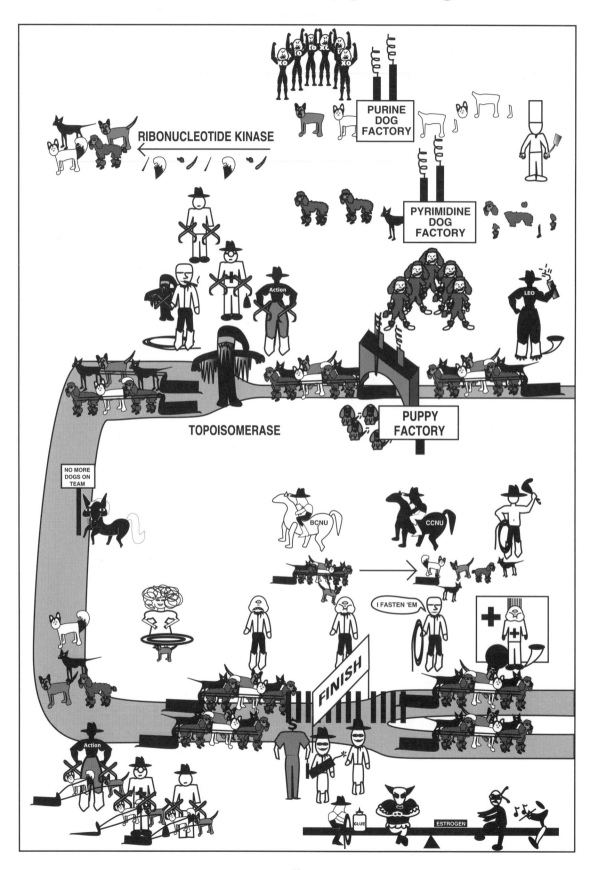

Picture Key

The difference between a normal cell and a neoplastic cell is subtle, although their effects are not. This difference is the rate of proliferation. Because of this, the main target for cancer cells has become the machinery for replication of the cell. As seen in the picture in the Introduction and antiviral section of this chapter, the life cycle of the cell is represented by a dog race. The synthesis of ribonucleotides, DNA, RNA, proteins, and ultimately mitosis of the cell is shown in this race. In chemotherapy for cancer, the main idea is to stop this machinery. As such, the picture will depict ways to stop the dog race.

Because the picture is the same as those seen throughout this chapter, please refer to the Introduction for the picture key. Specific additions for cancer chemotherapy are shown below.

Antineoplastic agents

The cell is malignant and proliferating

Cell cycle: from mitosis to mitosis

$G_0 \Rightarrow$ cells can reversibly enter this phase or irreversibly as in maturation

$G_1 \Rightarrow$ function of the cells occur in this phase; mainly RNA and protein synthesis

$S \Rightarrow$ DNA synthesis occurs in preparation for mitosis

$G_2 \Rightarrow$ cell arranges itself in preparation for mitosis

$M \Rightarrow$ Mitosis

Differences between normal and cancer cells:

Normal cells $\Rightarrow$ The majority of cells are in G_0 of the cell cycle.

Benign cancer $\Rightarrow$ The majority of cells are in S, G_1, and M, although they do not spread or invade.

Malignant cancer $\Rightarrow$ The majority of cells are in S, G_1, and M and they do spread (metastasize) and invade surrounding tissue.

DNA precursors $\Rightarrow$ Proliferating cells require abundant DNA precursors.

Things that take dogs out of the race

Race after race is occuring, without rest

Normal race:

The dogs rest after their last race. They prepare themselves to race again.

The section of the race where the team is at the puppy factory

The section of the race where the dog team is separated into two teams and a new line of dogs is placed on each sled

The two teams race towards the finish line.

The finish line, when the final two dog teams go their separate ways and prepare to race again

Differences between normal races and accelerated races:

Normal races $\Rightarrow$ In most of the races, the dogs are resting instead of running toward the finish line.

Benign races $\Rightarrow$ Most of the dogs are running toward the finish line.

Malignant races $\Rightarrow$ Most of the dogs are running toward the finish line. These races are bad because they can cause damage to the areas of the Phunny Pharm in which they occur.

Food and things used to make dogs for the race $\Rightarrow$ If many races are occuring, a lot of food and things to make dogs are required for the race.

Chemotherapeutic Targets

In treating cancer, all of the cancer cells must be killed or stopped so they cannot return to proliferate.

Drugs can be cell-cycle specific:

DNA synthesis inhibitors $\Rightarrow$ S-phase

DNA analogs $\Rightarrow$ Please refer to the DNA and RNA Primer (page 53).

Microtubule inhibitors $\Rightarrow$ M-phase

Drugs can be cell-cycle nonspecific:

DNA alkylators that are better for slow-growing tumors

Hormonal regulation:

Some cancer cells may retain their response to hormones that their cells of origin had. This response may result in increased growth when the hormone is present; therefore, the target is to decrease the amount of hormone.

Ways to Stop the Race

Can stop races at different areas of the race:

Can stop the race where the dogs are made

Dog impersonators

The fence of small tubes that makes the two dog teams go their separate ways (i.e., to different new races)

Can stop the race at anytime during the race:

People that put things on the dogs such that the dogs will not work properly

Some dogs run faster when they hear harmonies:

Can stop the harmonies that are making the dogs run faster. This will make the dogs slow down.

Antibiotics Used vs. Cancer in General

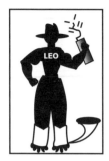

Bleomycin		**Big <u>Leo</u>, the First <u>Mycin</u> Brother**
mech	Reacts with DNA → hydrolysis to free bases	Big Leo blows up the dog team.
Tox	Lung and <u>skin</u> ⇒ pulmonary fibrosis and ulcerations	He <u>blows up</u> (sounds like "Bleo") lungs and skin (skin sounds like -my<u>cin</u>). He is also standing on tube from the Phunny Pharm Airport.‡

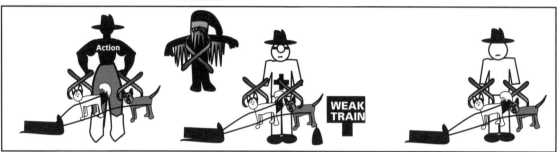

	Dactinomycin	**Doxorubicin**	**Daunorubicin**
N	<u>End in -mycin or -rubicin:</u> <u>Dactino</u>mycin <u>Dox</u>orubicin <u>Dauno</u>rubicin	<u>Mycin and Rubicin brothers:</u> <u>D-action</u> who deactivates the dog teams <u>Doc,</u> the first Rubicin brother <u>Dauno,</u> the second Rubicin brother	
mech	Intercalate into DNA between bases → inhibition of RNA and DNA synthesis. This intercalation also inhibits <u>topoisomerase</u> II → double strand breaks in DNA.	They have pinchers instead of hands, which they use to hold the two lines of dogs together; therefore, the two lines cannot separate, and other teams of dogs cannot be made from them. They also use the <u>top ice man of the race</u> to break up the dog team.	
Met	<u>Dox</u>orubicin ⇒ hepatic and biliary excretion	Doc Rubicin is a doctor ⇒ hepatic metabolism.*	
Tox	<u>Dactino</u>mycin ⇒ bone marrow depression, stomatitis, oral ulceration	<u>D-action</u> also deactivates the bone marrow.	
	<u>Dox</u>orubicin and <u>dauno</u>rubicin ⇒ cardiac → <u>congestive heart failure</u>, arrhythmias, pericarditis	<u>Doc</u> and <u>Dauno</u> Rubicin use pinchers to <u>weaken the Phunny Pharm Train</u>.†	
Rt	<u>Dactino</u>mycin ⇒ rapid IV <u>Dox</u>orubicin ⇒ IV		
Uses	<u>Dactino</u>mycin ⇒ <u>Wilms</u>' tumor, <u>testicular</u> cancer, <u>chorio</u>carcinoma <u>Dox</u>orubicin ⇒ maybe endless <u>Dauno</u>rubicin ⇒ acute <u>leuk</u>emias	Dactinomycin <u>will treat cancer</u>.	

---

*Rem: Virtually all "Docs" in the Phunny Pharm are hepatically metabolized.
†Rem: The heart is represented by the Phunny Pharm Train throughout the Phunny Pharm.
‡Rem: The lung is represented by the Phunny Pharm Airport throughout the Phunny Pharm.

Antimetabolites

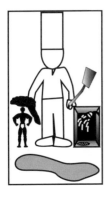

Methotrexate

N	Methotrexate	

mech Folic acid analog that irreversibly inhibits dihydrofolate reductase → depletion of intracellular dihydrofolate → shortage of purine nucleotides.
This is similar to the action of trimethoprim.
Sensitive cells are those that need a large amount of DNA precursors ⇒ those which are proliferating.

dist Large tissue distribution, including into any free water in the body.

Met Renal

Tox Free fluid, such as pleural effusion and ascites, are contraindications for use because methotrexate is distributed to these fluids.
Bone marrow depression, oral and GI ulceration, pulmonary infiltrates, hepatotoxicity
Nephrotoxicity that can be prevented with alkalinization

Uses Many uses
Must be used with leucovorin with high doses ⇒ a folinic acid to "rescue" normal cells from toxicity following a high dose of methotrexate.

Messes with Treats They Ate

A cook who messes with treats the dogs ate
The cook messes with the dying water foliage* → a shortage of purebreds (i.e., Alaskan Malamutes and German Shepherds)

The cook is a special friend of the goalie in the water polo game.†
The races that are vulnerable to this cook's attack are those that need a lot of treats for the purebred dogs because they are working hard.
This cook is a travelling cook.

He likes to go to the showers when he is through.

The cook likes to play in any free water such as the water on the runways at the Phunny Pharm Airport.

Lake of Vorin ⇒ a lake that has dying water foliage on it that can be eaten by the purebred dogs. This prepares them for the race.

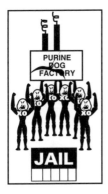

6-Mercaptopurine

N	6-Mercaptopurine	

mech Converted to an active form by enzymes of the salvage pathway
Ribonucleotides inhibit first step of purine nucleotide biosynthesis.

Inhibits conversion of IMP → GMP and AMP

6 Merciful People Capture Purebreds

6 merciful people capture purebreds and take them out of the race. They are "merciful" because they keep the dogs from working hard in the neoplastic races.

The six merciful people keep purebred dogs from being made, so they cannot be used in the neoplastic race.

---

*Note that the dying water foliage represents dihydrofolate reductase because the two sound alike.
†Rem: Trimethoprim is represented by the water polo goalie, as seen in the antimicrobial chapter—sulfonamides.

Met	Hepatic	The six merciful people are taken away by the police to the jail.*
	Xanthine oxidase inactivates it within the cell.	They have "XO" on their shirts.
Tox	Bone marrow depression and hepatotoxicity	The six people may hurt the police as the police try to stop them.
Uses	Acute lymphocytic leukemia	

Pyrimidine Antagonist

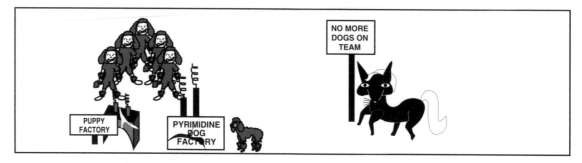

5-Fluorouracil

N	5-Fluorouracil (5-FU)
	Cytosine arabinoside (cytarabine, Ara-C)
mech	5-Fluorouracil ⇒ converted to ribonucleotide by salvage pathway → incorporated into RNA → inhibition of RNA function.
	Also → inhibits thymidylate synthetase → shortage of dTMP for synthesis of DNA
	Cytosine arabinoside ⇒ incorporated into DNA, inhibits DNA polymerase → inhibits DNA synthesis
Tox	Both ⇒ diarrhea, bone marrow depression
	5-Fluorouracil ⇒ oral and GI ulcers
	Cytosine arabinoside ⇒ CNS (cerebellar and ocular) and fever
Uses	5-Fluorouracil ⇒ GI, head and neck, breast and ovarian malignancies
	Cytosine arabinoside ⇒ leukemia and lymphoma

Cytosine Arabinoside

5 of your silly Toy Poodle imposters.

An Arabian coyote, he is a coyote impersonator who is a "sight to have seen."

5 of your silly Toy Poodle imposters get into the puppy factory and keep the runts from doing their job.

They also prevent production of the Toy Poodles that it needs for the race.

The Arabian coyote gets put on the dog team, and then prevents further dogs from getting on the team.

DNA Damaging Drugs

Alkylating Agents in General

N	Nitrogen mustards
	Mechlorethamine = nitrogen mustard
	Cyclophosphamide
	Ifosfamide
	Chlorambucil

Cowboys Who Tie the Dogs

The Cyclops†

Cyclops Clor who is a mean cowboy

Cyclops who fixes 'em to one another

I fasten 'em

Cyclops who drives an ambulance and tapes 'em together

---

*Rem: The liver is represented by the jail throughout the Phunny Pharm.
†Rem: Most drugs in the Phunny Pharm that have "chlor" in them are cyclops.

	Nitrosoureas		The night ropers
	Methylnitrosoureas		The cyclops night roper
	2-Chloroethylnitrosureas		Two cyclops night ropers
	Streptozotocin		A cowboy stripper who tosses his rope and
			tows the German Shepherd in
mech	Alkylate DNA at guanine bases ≡ transfer of		They all put things on the German Shepherds
	an active alkyl group to DNA. The alkyl		that connect them to other dogs on the team →
	group cross-links and breaks DNA chains.		the team to fall apart.
Phase	Cell-cycle nonspecific		They can get the dog team at any time.
Uses	Slow-growing tumors, since these drugs are		These are best at getting the dogs in the slower
	cell nonspecific		races.

Nitrogen Mustards

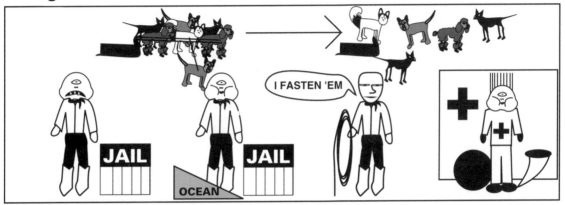

	Mechlorethamine	Cyclophosphamide	Ifosfamide	Chlorambucil

N	Nitrogen mustards		The Cyclops
	Mechlorethamine = nitrogen mustard		Cyclops named Clor who is a mean cowboy
	Cyclophosphamide		Cyclops who fixes 'em to one another
	Ifosfamide		I fasten 'em
	Chlorambucil		Cyclops named Clor who drives an
			ambulance and tapes 'em together
mech	Alkylate DNA		They all put something on the German
			Shepherds that connects them to other dogs
			on the team → the team to fall apart.
	Cyclophosphamide ⇒ essentially a cyclic		"Cyclo" who fixes 'em to one another enters the
	derivative of mechlorethamine, allowing it		Phunny Pharm through the ocean.* He is
	to have an oral route of administration. It		processed by the police† and then is allowed
	requires enzymatic activation by the P-450		to fasten the German Shepherds to other dogs.
	system to "de-cycle it."		
Tox	All ⇒ secondary malignancies (e.g., AML),		The person in the sled must drink a lot. If he
	bone marrow suppression, nausea and		does not, his bladder will become bloody.
	vomiting, alopecia, and sterility in men		All the cyclops are bald except the ambulance
	Cyclophosphamide and ifosfamide ⇒		driver.
	hemorrhagic cystitis (prevented with fluids)		
	and SIADH		
	Chlorambucil ⇒ no alopecia, pulmonary		This cyclops has hair, but is stepping on a tube
	infiltrates and fibrosis		from the Phunny Pharm Airport.
Rt	Cyclophosphamide ⇒ PO- or IV-activated		"Cyclo" came from the ocean.
	on the first pass through the liver		
	Chlorambucil ⇒ PO		"Chlor" ⇒ "oral"

*Rem: The ocean represents the GI tract throughout The Phunny Pharm.
†Rem: Police or referees represent the liver throughout The Phunny Pharm.

Phase   Cell-cycle nonspecific
Uses   Breast, lymphomas, Hodgkin's, ovarian, acute
         lymphocytic leukemia, lung malignancies

Nitrosoureas in General   The Night Ropers

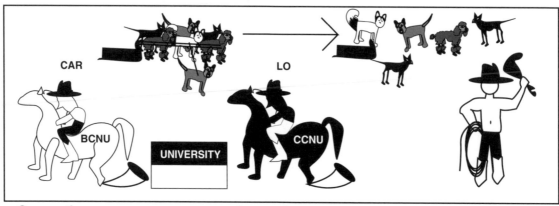

Carmustine	Lomustine	Streptozotocin
N 2-Chloroethylnitrosureas: end in -<u>mustine</u> <u>Car</u>mustine (BCNU) <u>Lo</u>mustine (CCNU)	Two cowboys who ride a <u>mustang</u>. Their names together are <u>Car-Lo</u> ⇒ Car-Lo the mustang riders. They also have their nicknames on their mustangs (i.e., BCNU or CCNU).	

<u>Strep</u>tozotocin	A cowboy <u>strip</u>per who <u>tosses</u> his rope and <u>tows</u> the dog <u>in</u>.	
mech Decompose to <u>DNA</u> alkylators	They all put <u>things</u> on the German Shepherds that connect them to other dogs on the team → the team to fall apart.	
Dist Crosses blood–<u>brain</u> barrier	They can sneak into the <u>University</u>.*	
Tox Carmustine and lomustine ⇒ severe bone marrow suppression that can be delayed up to 6 wk before onset, nausea, pulmonary fibrosis.	The person in the sled gets sick to his stomach. Car-Lo are standing on a tube from the Phunny Pharm Airport.	
Uses <u>Car</u>mustine and <u>Lo</u>mustine ⇒ <u>brain</u> tumors because they cross BBB; lymphomas and melanoma	<u>Car-Lo</u> can get into the <u>University</u>.	
<u>Strep</u>tozotocin ⇒ pancreatic <u>islet</u> cell tumor ⇒ streptozotocin has affinity for these cells	He loves to strip on an <u>island</u>.	

Nonalkylating Agent that Causes Cross-Linking of DNA

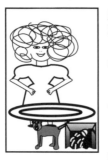

	Cisplatin	My Sis' Who Plates Them
N	<u>Cisplatin</u>	My <u>sis'</u>, who puts a <u>plate</u> on the German Shepherds
mech	Cross-linking of DNA at <u>guanine</u> bases	My sis' puts a <u>plate</u> on the German Shepherds that locks them to other dogs on the team.
Tox	<u>Renal</u> tubular dysfunction → severe K and Mg wasting, nausea, peripheral neuropathy, and ototoxicity.	She destroys the <u>showers</u>.
Uses	Ovarian lung, lymphomas, head and neck, and testicular malignancies	

---

*Rem: University represents the CNS throughout <u>The Phunny Pharm</u>.

Vinca Alkaloids and Taxol

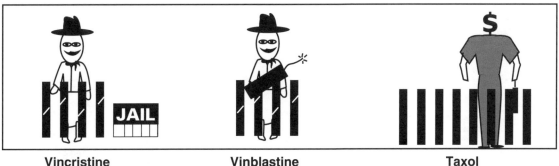

	Vincristine	**Vinblastine**	**Taxol**

N	Vinca alkaloids begin with <u>Vin:</u>
	   Vin<u>cristine</u>
	   Vin<u>blastine</u>
	   Taxol
		The <u>Vin</u> sisters:
		   <u>Christine</u>
		   <u>Blasting</u>
		<u>Tax</u> person who taxes everything (<u>all</u>) but fences

mech	All inhibit microtubules → inhibition of mitosis and other cellular processes. Vinca alkaloids disrupt microtubule formation. Taxol promotes microtubule formation.	They destroy the fence that makes the two dog teams go their separate ways (i.e., to different new races). The tax person does not tax fences because she promotes the building of this fence.
Met	Vinca alkaloids ⇒ hepatic	The sisters are stopped by the police.
Tox	Vinca alkaloids → alopecia, paralytic ileus Vin<u>cristine</u> ⇒ peripheral neuropathy, but **No** bone marrow suppression <u>Vinblastine bone</u> ⇒ marrow suppression is limiting factor in use <u>Taxol</u> ⇒ marrow suppression and sensory neuropathy	They are both bald. She doesn't touch bones; she lets her sister, Blasting, blast the bones. Blasting Vin blasts the <u>bones</u> of the person in the sled with a tube of dynamite.
Rt	IV	
Uses	<u>Taxol</u> ⇒ ovarian carcinoma	

Etoposide

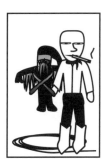

Etoposide (VP16–213)		**Ernie Hits <u>Top</u> Ice Man's <u>Side</u>**
mech	Interferes with topoisomerase II → double-stranded breaks in DNA	Ernie hits <u>top ice man's side</u> → the dogs to fall off of the sled
Tox	Bone marrow suppression, anaphylaxis, alopecia, mucositis, hypotension	Ernie is bald.
Rt	IV or PO	
Uses	Testicular and lung cancers	Ernie had some Rocky Mountain oysters for dinner and enjoyed a "roll 'yer own" (a cigarette).

Sex Hormones in General

Some of the chemotherapy for cancer that originates from cells that are stimulated by sex hormones is somewhat unique. This stimulation can be removed by medications. Even though this will not eliminate the neoplastic cells, it can prevent them from growing and causing problems. Estrogen stimulates some breast cancer to grow, and decreasing the amount of estrogen can slow growth of the neoplasm. In the same respect, testosterone increases the growth of prostate cancer, and proliferation of this cancer can be slowed by decreasing the testosterone.

It is easiest to consider estrogen as the complete opposite of testosterone. Estrogen has the opposite effects of testosterone, which implies that ⇒ estrogen slows growth of prostate cancer and that testosterone slows growth of breast cancer. Therefore, the following picture puts these drugs on a see-saw. Estrogen is on one end and testosterone is on the other end of the see-saw. If the drug is an antagonist, then it is shown on the opposite side of the see-saw.

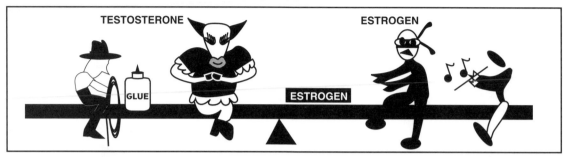

Aminoglutethimide	Tamoxifen	Estrogen	Leuprolide	Flutamide

N — Estrogen antagonists:
    Aminoglutethimide

    Tamoxifen
  Testosterone antagonists: (ELF)
    Estrogen

    Leuprolide
    Flutamide

Things on the testosterone side of the see-saw:
    A minor drug that glues and tethers the remaining estrogen
    Tammy the ox
Things on the estrogen side of the see-saw:
    ¢: Not pictured in the picture, except as the words
    Loopy prowler
    A flutist

mech — Estrogen antagonists:
    Aminoglutethimide ⇒ eliminates the adrenal source of estrogen
    Tamoxifen ⇒ estrogen receptor antagonist

  Testosterone inhibitors:
    Estrogen

    Leuprolide ⇒ nonsurgical orchiectomy
      LHRH agonist → ↓ gonadotropin → ↓ testosterone production
    Flutamide ⇒ testosterone receptor antagonist

Things on the testosterone side of the see-saw:
    A minor drug that glues and tethers the remaining estrogen
    Tammy the ox sits on the testosterone side and weighs it down → decreased estrogen effects.
Things on the estrogen side of the see-saw:
    ¢: Not pictured in the picture except as the words
    Loopy prowler has a shirt that says, "LHRH." He is on the estrogen side of the see-saw → ↓ testosterone.
    A flutist who sits on the estrogen side and plays music → ↓ testosterone effects.

Tox — Estrogen ⇒ gynecomastia, edema, sexual impotence, thromboembolism, deep venous thrombosis

    ¢: These are some of the actions of estrogen

The Autonomic Nervous System

Life is not easy, but the organization of our nervous system takes a tremendous load off our minds. It is ingeniously separated into the autonomic nervous system (ANS) and the central nervous system (CNS). The ANS hides the maintenance of the body's normal functions from the conscious awareness of these activities by the CNS. Fortunately (or unfortunately), this allows the CNS to concern itself with more important things like pharmacology.

The ANS is further divided into two largely opposing branches: the parasympathetic nervous system (PNS) and the sympathetic nervous system (SNS). These systems control the gastrointestinal tract, cardiovascular system, lungs, genitals, and urinary tract; protect the eyes; and regulate body temperature. In general, they are separated anatomically and functionally, and the action occuring in the organ is a result of the **balance** between the two.

Functions of ANS

In general, the two branches of the ANS have opposite actions, yet they may work together for some things (such as sexual function) or complement the action of the other (as in perspiration). The PNS is concerned with the day-to-day activities of ensuring that the body has enough energy and is protected. The SNS is usually thought of as the "fight or flight" response, because it is responsible for taking over the body and getting us off our duffs in times of stress. Thank goodness, the **balance** between the two usually lies in favor of the PNS, which allows us to hang out and be couch potatoes instead of fighting or fleeing.

The following table reviews the actions of each system and emphasizes in **bold** type the system that predominates in the resting state. Become familiar with it now, but keep in mind that we will return to it with some memory help later.

	PNS (5 P's + . . .)	SNS (5 S's + . . .)
Eyes	**Miosis** (pinpoint)	Mydriasis (dilate)
	Accomodation	Distant vision
Mouth	**Salivation**	
GI tract	**Increases motility**	Decreases motility
	Secretion of acid, pancreatic enzymes	Inhibits secretion and inhibits insulin release
	Relaxation of sphincters	Contraction of sphincters (sphincter)
	Contraction of gallbladder	Relaxation of gallbladder
	Defecation (poop)	
Respiratory tract	Constriction of bronchi	Dilation of bronchi
	Increases respiratory secretions	
	Increases beating of cilia	
Heart	**Decreases chronotropy**	Increases chronotropy
	Decreases inotropy	Increases inotropy (stronger)
Genitals	Erection (point)	Ejaculation (shoot)
Urinary tract	**Urination** (pee)	Retention (stop)
Arterioles	Dilatation	**Constriction**
Veins	None	**Constriction**
Sweat glands	Generalized sweat (perspire)	**Localized sweat** (sweat)

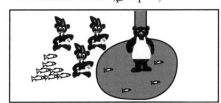 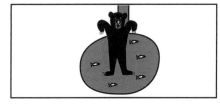

ANS General Organization

In general, all efferent nerve pathways involve two nerves extending from the CNS to the target organ. This includes the parasympathetic and sympathetic pathways, as well as the corticospinal tract to skeletal muscle.

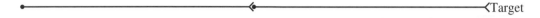

In the corticospinal tract, the synapse occurs in the anterior horn of the spinal cord. In the ANS, a ganglion separates the two nerves; therefore, the first can be designated "preganglionic" and the second "postganglionic." Because the nerves synapse at the ganglia, they can also be referred to as pre- and postsynaptic.

presynaptic nerve   postsynaptic nerve
●————————————————◎————————————————<Target
                              ganglion

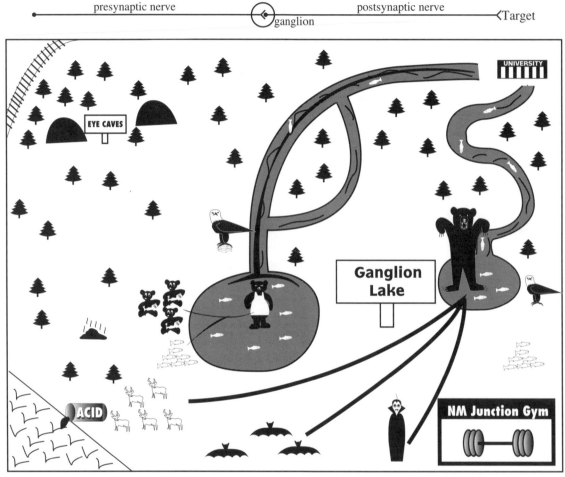

Picture Key

This picture takes us to the The Phunny Pharm Forest, where the female bear fishes and takes her catch to her cubs or another bear may scare some animals.

Preganglionic nerve	The river that flows into the lake
The ganglion	The lake
Acetylcholine	The ace fish
Cholinergic receptor	The bear or cubs who take the fish
Muscarinic cholinergic receptor	The three musketeer cubs
Nicotinic cholinergic receptor	Nicky the momma bear or Nick the mean old grizzly bear
Binding of acetylcholine to receptor at the ganglia	The bears catch fish from the lake.
Acetylcholine esterase	Ester the eagle, who catches the fish before the bears or the cubs can get them

Parasympathetic:	**Nicky the bear taking fish to her cubs:**
Postganglionic nerve	Nicky the bear as she returns to the cubs
Binding of acetylcholine to receptor at the target organ; note that this is the muscarinic receptor	The three musketeer cubs get the fish from their mother

Target organs	Things the cubs can do after they eat the fish
Postganglionic parasympathetic nerves are short	The cubs remain relatively close to Nicky.
Sympathetic:	**Nick the bear scaring the antelope and bats:**
Postganglionic nerve	Nick the grizzly bear's journey to the antelope or bats after eating the fish
<u>Norepinephrine</u>	The <u>nor epi cross</u>, which Nick uses to scare antelope and bats
Adrenergic receptor	Antelope and bats that Nick scares
Binding of epinephrine to receptor at the target organ	Nick scaring the antelope and bats
Target organs for sympathetics	Things the antelope and bats do after they are scared
Postganglionic sympathetic nerves are long	The antelope and bats are a long distance from Nick's ganglion lake
Neuromuscular junction	NM junction gym

Comparisons Between Branches of ANS

Parasympathetic Nervous System In the Phunny Pharm

Preganglionic nerve is long and extends to the target organ.

This river from the University is long, and it forms a lake that is near the target organs.

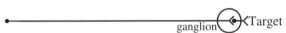

Preganglionic to postganglionic nerve ratio is 1:1.

Nicky the bear has only one set of cubs, and after eating the fish, the cubs can do only one thing.

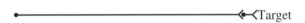

Local ganglionic synapse and 1:1 distribution allows for fine control of function of the target organ.

¢

Sympathetic Nervous System

Preganglionic nerve is short and extends to a ganglia distant from the target organ.

In the Phunny Pharm

The river from the University is short, and it forms a lake that is far from the target organs such that once Nick eats a fish, he must walk a long distance before he can scare the antelope and bats.

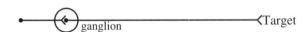

Pre:post is 1:many ⇒ up to 1,000s.

Nick the bear can scare thousands of antelope and bats at once.

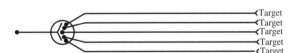

Distance between target organ and ganglia and extensive signal distribution of a small number of nerves (i.e., ramification of signal) allow for a more generalized action at times of "fight or flight."

¢

Signal Transmission

The delivery of the signal from the brain to the target organ occurs in several steps. The first is simply the transmission of the action potential from the brain to the ganglia via the preganglionic nerve axon. The second major step is the transmission of the impulse from the preganglionic nerve to the postganglionic nerve. Third, the action potential begins in the second nerve and is carried down this postganglionic nerve axon. Finally, the action potential is transmitted from the postganglionic nerve to the target organ and an action occurs.

The most important steps to the pharmacology of this system occur in the transmission of the action potential from preganglionic nerve to postganglionic nerve at the ganglia and transmission from the postganglionic nerve to the target organ. This is due to the fact that except for local administration of drugs to a nerve axon, the movement of an action potential down an axon is inaccessible to pharmacology. In contrast, the synapses allow easier targets for manipulation by drugs.

Signal Transmission Across the Synaptic Cleft

The *italicized* steps that follow are those that are *not* readily accessible to pharmacologic intervention.

1. *The action potential arrives at the presynaptic membrane.*
2. Influx of Ca^{2+} occurs and neurotransmitter is **released** into the synaptic cleft.
3. Neurotransmitter evades postsynaptic enzymes and **binds** to receptors at the postsynaptic membrane → an action potential in a postsynaptic nerve, or an "action" in a postsynaptic cell.

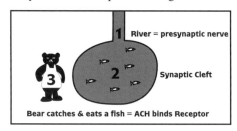

Signal Termination in the Synaptic Cleft

The *italicized* steps that follow are those that are *not* readily accessible to pharmacologic intervention. Please note that for the SNS, neurotransmitter catabolism is not important in the synaptic cleft.

Parasympathetic

1. Neurotransmitter can be catabolized by a postsynaptic enzyme.
2. Neurotransmitter can be taken up by the presynaptic cell.
3. *Neurotransmitter can diffuse away from the synapse.*

Sympathetic:

1. Neurotransmitter is taken up by the presynaptic cell.
2. *Neurotransmitter can diffuse away from the synapse.*

As can be seen from the preceding summary, drugs can be used to increase or decrease the transmission of signal from the brain to the target organ by interfering at the appropriate location. Before we explore this subject further, more of the anatomy and physiology must be learned.

Neurotransmitters and Receptors

As outlined previously, the neurotransmitters and their receptors play an integral part in ensuring that the signal gets from the brain to the target organ. In addition, they also help to delineate a difference between the action of the PNS and the SNS that allows us to manipulate one or the other preferentially. This difference lies in the neurotransmitter that is used in the synapse between the **postganglionic nerve and the target organ**. For the PNS, this is acetylcholine and for the SNS, norepinephrine.

Although this seems easy enough, the "neurotransmitters and receptors" of the ANS are very difficult concepts to keep straight. One problem with this topic is that the organization often exists only in an abstract form. Personally, I could not picture this organization in my mind's eye. Instead, I tried to memorize the locations of receptors by words like "postganglionic" and "preganglionic," even though they had no physical meaning to me (pretty dumb, but I am not alone). So take a minute now to look back at your anatomy book and visualize the location of autonomic ganglia and the organization that is reviewed above.

Now remember that both sympathetic and parasympathetic nerves synapse in a ganglia before proceeding on their way to the target organ as the postganglionic nerve.

Now, the Laws of Two's

There are two classes of neurotransmitter in the ANS:

Cholinergic $\Rightarrow$ acetylcholine (Ach)
Adrenergic* $\Rightarrow$ norepinephrine (Norepi)[†]
There are two classes of cholinergic receptors[‡]:
   Nicotinic
   Muscarinic
There are two types of adrenergic receptors:
   α
   β
There are two types of each adrenergic receptor:
   α_1 and α_2

   β_1 and β_2

Two things are caught or carried by Nick and Nicky:
   Ace fish
   Nor epi cross

Nicky and Nick the bears at Ganglion Lake
The three musketeer cubs
Nick scares two types of animals:
   Antelope
   Bats and vampires

The two types of receptors will only be differentiated by the location in which the antelope are scared.
Vampire and bats

Location of Receptors

Cholinergic Receptors:

Nicotinic Receptor

Muscarinic Receptor
Adrenergic Receptors α & β

All ganglia and parasympathetic end-organ innervation
The ganglionic receptor, certain areas of the brain, and neuromuscular junction[§]
The parasympathetic end-organ receptor
Sympathetic end-organ innervation

Pharmacologic Targets

One can arrive at the targets accessible to pharmacologic intervention if one understands the physiology presented above. For example, to increase transmission at the target organ, you must envision ways to increase the amount of neurotransmitter seen by the postsynaptic receptors at the target organ: by blocking enzymatic cleavage of the neurotransmitter, by blocking reuptake of neurotransmitter by presynaptic cell, or by mimicking the action of the neurotransmitter with a drug.

---

*Note: This class is called adrenergic because epinephrine = adrenaline and norepinephrine = noradrenaline.
[†]Please note that this class is also called "catecholamines." It is imperative that you don't get these confused with acetylcholine (i.e., catecholamine ≠ acetylcholine).
[‡]Rem: A cholinergic receptor responds to acetylcholine and an adrenergic receptor responds to an adrenergic neurotransmitter.
[§]Please note that the neuromuscular junction is the synapse between somatic motor nerves and voluntary muscles. This topic will be discussed again.

Parasympathetic Nervous System

As seen in the Introduction to the autonomic nervous system, the sites of pharmacologic intervention occur at the synapse between the pre- and postganglionic nerves and the postganglionic synapse with the target organ.

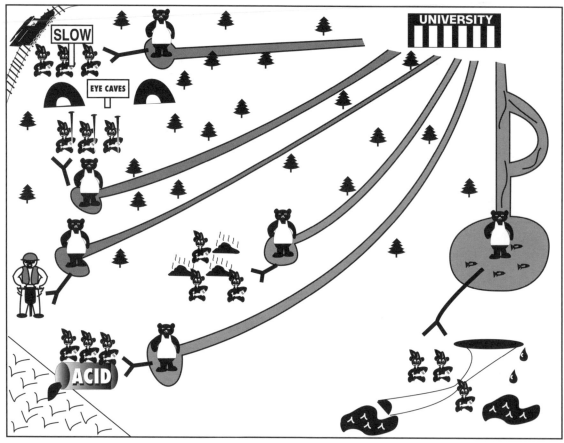

Picture Key

The picture for the parasympathetic nervous system only focuses upon Nicky and her three musketeer cubs. To review:

Cholinergic receptor
   Nicotinic cholinergic receptor
   Muscarinic cholinergic receptor
Binding of acetylcholine to receptor at the ganglia
Postganglionic nerve
Binding of acetylcholine to receptor at the target organ

Acetylcholine esterase

Target organ effects of parasympathetic nerve
   stimulation

The bear or cubs when they take the fish
   Nicky the bear
   The three musketeer cubs
Nicky the bear catches a fish from the lake.
Nicky the bear as she returns to the cubs
The three musketeer cubs get the fish from their
   mother, and then do what bear cubs do.
Ester the eagle, who catches the fish before
   Nicky or the cubs can get them
Things the three musketeer cubs do after they
   eat the fish from their mother

More Picture Keys

The actions of the PNS can be remembered by visualizing the actions of the three musketeer cubs actions after they eat the fish from their mom Nicky. The actions represent associations that will be used throughout The Phunny Pharm.

	PNS Action	**In the Phunny Pharm**
Eyes	**Miosis** (pinpoint)	The three musketeer cubs hold a pin and the eye cave is closed.
	Accommodation	
Mouth	**Salivation**	The cubs salivate*when they see the fish.
GI tract	**Increase motility**	After they eat, they go swimming in the ocean and make the water churn.
	Secretion of acid, pancreatic enzymes	After they eat, they release acid into the ocean.
	Relaxation of sphincters	
	Contraction of gall bladder	
	Defecation (poop)	They poop in the woods.
Respiratory tract	Constriction of bronchi	The three musketeer cubs squeeze the tunnels to the airports.
	Respiratory secretions	They make it rain at the airport.
	Increased beating of cilia	
Heart	**Decrease chronotropy**	The three musketeer cubs slow the train and make it weaker.
	Decrease inotropy	
Genitals	Erection (point)	(Skip this one, thank you very much).
Urinary tract	**Urination** (pee)	The cubs must wear diapers (i.e., Pampers) because they have not been potty trained.
Arterioles	Dilatation	The cubs like to play "highway workers" ⇒ they make more roads.
Veins	None	The cubs do not like to play in the parking lot, because nothing is happening there.
Sweat glands	Generalized sweat (perspire)	**They play so hard, they perspire.**

---

* Note: Not one of the "S's" of the sympathetic actions.

Parasympathomimetics: Things that Increase the Amount of Fish for the Bears and Cubs

To get parasympathetic effects when giving a medication, the drug must **increase** the "effective" amount of acetylcholine (Ach) present in the synapse. This can first be accomplished by giving a drug that diffuses into the synapses and acts like acetylcholine (i.e., binds and stimulates the cholinergic receptor). This example is an **acetylcholine receptor agonist.** The second way the amount of Ach can be increased is to inhibit the degradation of acetylcholine present in the synapse by blocking the acetylcholinesterase (i.e., **acetylcholine esterase inhibitor**).

Please notice that Ach could be increased by other methods such as increasing its release from the presynaptic membrane or inhibiting the diffusion of Ach from the synapse. Although these methods exist, they are **not** utilized to obtain parasympathomimetic effects.

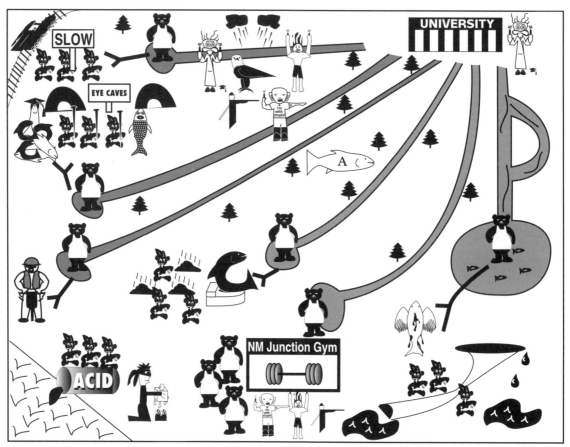

Picture Key

Binding of acetylcholine to muscarinic cholinergic receptor at the target organ

The three musketeer cubs get the fish from their mother Nicky.

Target organ action when stimulated by PNS
Acetylcholinesterase
Pupillary response to muscarinic cholinergic stimulation
   Constriction = miosis = pinpoint
PNS mimetic is accomplished by blocking Ach esterase
   or by mimicking <u>Ach</u>.

The things the cubs do after they eat the fish.
Ester the eagle, who takes fish from the cubs
The three musketeer cubs are holding a <u>pin</u> ⇒
   pinpoint pupils and saying, "Oh my oses!"
Cubs can get more fish by blocking Ester the
   eagle or by giving them fish that are similar
   to <u>Ace</u> the fish.

Direct-Acting Cholinergic Receptor Agonists in General

N   <u>Ace</u>tylcholine
         <u>Beth</u>anechol
         <u>Carba</u>chol
         <u>Pilocarp</u>ine
         <u>Me</u>thacholine

Tox   Should not be used in people with:
         Asthma ⇒ ↑ bronchoconstriction
         Peptic ulcer disease ⇒ ↑ acid production
         Cardiac disease ⇒ ↓ inotropy and
            chronotropy
         Parkinson's disease ⇒ may get ↑ rigidity
         Hyperthyroidism ⇒ ↑ risk of atrial fibrillation

<u>Ace</u>, the main fish
<u>Beth</u>any, the bathroom fish
Fish with armor of <u>carbu</u>ncles
<u>Pile of carps</u>
<u>Me</u>ssy, the flying fish
¢

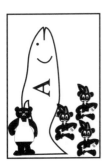

Acetylcholine

mech   Rapid hydrolysis by <u>acety</u>choline,
       <u>esterase</u>, and plasma,
       pseudocholinesterases
       Ach would, if it were not hydrolyzed,
       bind and activate all cholinergic
       receptors. This includes nicotinic
       and muscarinic.

Uses   Not used secondary to rapid hydrolysis
       and nonspecificity of actions

Ace, the Main Fish

<u>Ester the Eagle</u> catches Ace very
     easily.

Eaten by both Nicky and the three
     musketeer cubs

Because Ace would be eaten quickly
     by Ester, it is not used.

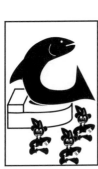

Bethanechol

N   <u>Beth</u>anechol

mech   Relatively selective for <u>musc</u>arinic
       receptors of the GI and urinary
       tracts

Dist   Does not penetrate into the CNS
Rt   <u>PO</u> (poorly absorbed), and
       subcutaneous only

Uses   Prevents urinary retention and
       inadequate emptying of bladder
       Should not be used if urinary
       obstruction is present

Bethany, the Bathroom Fish

<u>Beth</u>any, the <u>bath</u>room fish, who
     makes the cubs poop and pee after
     they eat
Makes the three <u>musketeer</u> cubs poop
     and pee, but Nicky the Bear does
     not eat these fish (i.e., does not bind
     nicotinic receptors)
Bethany is not wearing a mortarboard.
The cubs <u>eat</u> Bethany.

Bethany helps the cubs to poop and
     pee.

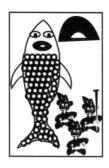

Carbachol

mech	Stimulates mostly <u>muscarinic</u> receptors
Met	<u>Resistant</u> to acetylcholinesterase
Rt	Intraophthalmic only
Uses	Glaucoma, and to produce miosis in ocular surgery

Fish with Armor of <u>Carbuncles</u>

Can be eaten by the three <u>musketeer</u> cubs

Armor of carbuncles <u>protects</u> it from Ester the eagle.

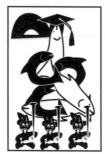

Pilo<u>carp</u>ine

mech	Mainly stimulates muscarinic receptors
	Tertiary amine, therefore → CNS stimulation
Rt	Mainly intraophthalmic
Uses	Glaucoma

Pile of Carps

The pile of carps are mainly eaten by the three musketeer cubs.

These fish are wearing mortarboards ⇒ get into CNS.

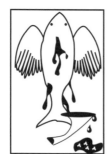

Methacholine

Rt	Inhalation
Uses	"Methacholine challenge" ⇒ diagnosis of bronchial hyperreactivity.

<u>Messy</u>, the Flying Fish

This is a flying fish.*

The flying fish close the tubes to the airport → ↓ in the number of planes flying into the airport

Cholinesterase Inhibitors

Reversible Cholinesterase Inhibitors in General

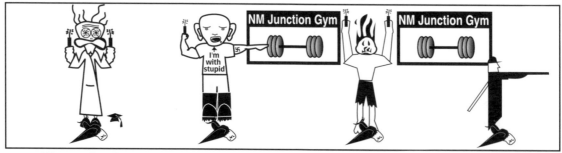

	Physostigmine	**Neostigmine**	**Pyridostigmine**	**Edrophonium**

N	End in-<u>stigmine</u>		People that block Ester the eagle with <u>sticks of dynamite</u>:
	<u>Phys</u>ostigmine		Mad <u>phys</u>icist with <u>sticks of dynamite</u>
	<u>Neo</u>stigmine		The <u>neo</u>-Nazi with <u>sticks of dynamite</u>
	<u>Pyr</u>idostigmine		<u>Pyr</u>omaniac with <u>sticks of dynamite</u> who <u>rids</u> the lake of eagles
	Ed<u>rophon</u>ium		<u>Ed</u> is a <u>phony</u> decoy of an eagle hunter that keeps Ester away.
mech	Block <u>acetylcholinesterase</u> reversibly → a ↓ in metabolism of Ach → ↑ duration of action of Ach → ↑ stimulation of cholinergic receptors		They throw sticks of dynamite to <u>Ester the eagle</u>, that blow her up → ↑ number of fish for the bears to take out of the lake.

---

*Rem: All things that fly in the Phunny Pharm can be administered by aerosol.

Dist	Physostigmine is a tertiary amine ⇒ gets into the CNS.	The mad physicist is the only one who has a college education ⇒ He wears a mortarboard.
	Neostigmine and pyridostigmine are quaternary amines ⇒ have a preferential action at the <u>neuromuscular junction,</u> because they do not penetrate into the fat surounding the autonomic ganglia. They also do not get into the CNS.	The <u>neo</u>-Nazi and the <u>pyro</u>maniac mainly act at the <u>NM Junction Gym</u>. They are flexing their biceps. They do not have a mortarboard.
	Edrophonium is also a quaternary amine ⇒ does not get into brain.	Ed is not wearing a mortarboard; he has a hunting cap.
$t_{1/2}$	Edrophonium ⇒ very short	The phony decoy only works for a short time.
Rt	Edrophonium ⇒ IV	
Uses	All can be used for treatment or diagnosis of myasthenia gravis ⇒ ↓ metabolism of Ach → ↑ duration of action of Ach → ↑ stimulation of cholinergic receptors at the neuromuscular junction	They are **all** flexing their biceps. They are actually preventing the eagles from eating the fish → leaves more for Nicky when she goes to the NM Junction Gym.
	Because only nicotinic effects are desired in treating myasthenia gravis, muscarinic side effects can be ↓ with <u>atropine.</u>	<u>The trap in the pines</u> can prevent the cubs from going crazy from the extra fish, when the eagles are gone. The <u>trap in the pines</u> prevents Nicky the bear from taking too many fish to the cubs.
	Physostigmine ⇒ glaucoma	
	Neostigmine ⇒ atony of detrusor muscle of bladder, paralytic ileus, and atony of GI tract	
	Edrophonium ⇒ "<u>tensilon test</u>": Diagnosis of myasthenia gravis ⇒ Give the patient edrophonium and if strength improves ⇒ the patient has myastenia gravis.	The phony decoy is made of <u>tinfoil</u>. Ed is flexing his biceps.

Irreversible Cholinesterase Inhibitors

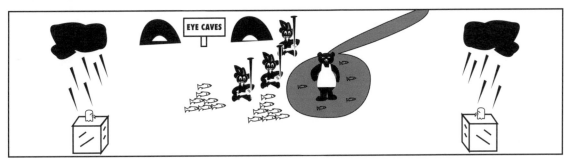

	Isoflurophate	**Echothiophate**
N	<u>Iso</u>flurophate	<u>Ice</u> storm that <u>flew</u> in
	<u>Echo</u>thiophate	<u>Echo</u> of the ice storm that flew in; it flew in <u>late</u>. This is a mirror image of the picture for isoflurophate.
mech	Covalent phosphorylation with cholinesterase that cannot be broken. This irreversibility takes about 30 minutes.	The ice storm freezes Ester the eagle so she cannot take fish from the bears or the cubs.
	Only way to restore action of cholinesterase is by synthesis of new enzymes	The only way to get new Esters is for the eagle chicks to grow up.

Dist   Isoflurophate ⇒ moves across all membranes   The storm can fly anywhere it wants.
          Echothiophate ⇒ does not get into the CNS.
Tox   Prolonged use may → cataracts   It can freeze and crack the lens of your eye.
Uses   Glaucoma
          Nerve gas

Irreversible Acetylcholinesterase Antidote

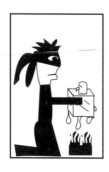

Pralidoxime   **A <u>Prowler</u> with a <u>Box</u> of <u>Pine</u>**

mech   Irreversible cholinesterase inhibitors   The prowler with a box of pine sets
          take time to form the covalent bond   the box on fire and thaws <u>Ester</u>
          with the enzyme and thereafter   before she gets to the point where
          become irreversible. Pralidoxime   she cannot recover from the ice
          has a higher affinity for the enzymes   storm's freeze ⇒ therefore, Ester
          and will displace the cholinesterase   can eat fish.
          inhibitor from the enzyme if given
          before bond formation.

Dist   Does not get into CNS   Prowler is not wearing a mortarboard.

Parasympatholytics: Things That Decrease the Amount of Fish the Bears and Cubs Eat

To get antiparasympathetic effects, the drug must **decrease** the amount of acetylcholine the receptors "see" in the synapse. The only way this can be accomplished with drugs is by inhibiting the acetylcholine receptor at the postsynaptic membrane of the ganglion or the target organ. It is important to review the effects of muscarinic blockade versus nicotinic blockade discussed in the parasympathetic Introduction.

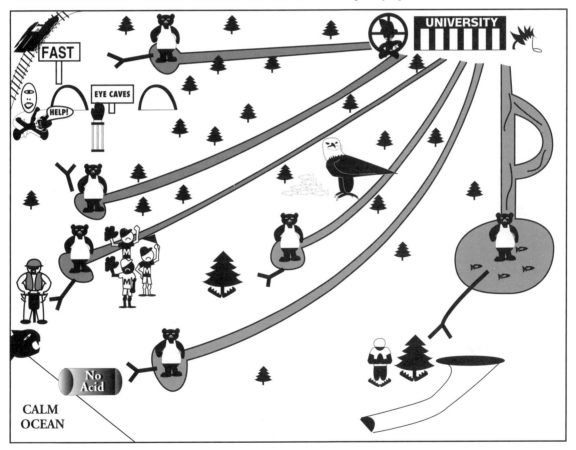

Picture Key

PNSolytic action is accomplished by preventing the binding of acetylcholine to muscarinic cholinergic receptors at the target organ.

Target organ action without stimulation by PNS.

Ganglionic blockade

The three musketeer cubs are trapped and cannot get the fish from their mother Nicky, and they cannot run around the phorest and get into mischief.

Things that are happening while the cubs are trapped

Stop Nicky from catching fish.

Antimuscarinics in General

N	Tertiary amines:	Things that get the three musketeer cubs:
	Atropine	<u>A trap</u> in the <u>pines</u>
	Scopolamine	Hunter's <u>scope</u> fixed on cub
	Benztropine	<u>Bent pine trap</u>
	Tertiary amines used only in ophthalmology:	
	Cyclopentolate	The <u>cyclop</u>s who eats cubs
	Tropicamide	<u>Trop</u>hy used to <u>pick</u> his <u>eye</u>
	Quaternary amines:	
	Ipratropium	<u>I pray to trap</u> 'em.
	Propantheline	<u>Prowling panther</u>

mech	Mainly block muscarinic cholinergic receptors by competitively binding the receptor and preventing activation	Things that get the three musketeer cubs and prevent them from taking the fish from Nicky the bear
	Decrease parasympathetic effects, such that sympathetics begin to predominate:	Block the three musketeer cubs from doing anything such that the effects of Nick the bear scaring animals will begin to dominate
	Eyes → mydriasis and cycloplegia	¢: These are opposite effects of muscarinic stimulation.
	Resp → bronchodilation and ↓ secretions	
	CV → ↑ heart rate	
	GI → ↓ salivation, ↓ motility, and ↓ acid secretion	
	GU → urine retention	
	Skin → anhidrosis (↓ sweating)	
Dist	Tertiary amines are well absorbed and distribute throughout the body, whereas quaternary amines infrequently cross membranes.	¢: Charged ions (i.e., quaternary amines) cross membranes less easily than uncharged ions.
Tox	Extension of above parasympatholytic effects	¢: More of the same effects
	CNS → restlessness, hallucinations, ataxia	
Uses	Used when above actions are desired	¢: From mechanism of action
	Prevent bradycardia in surgery	
	Prevent muscarinic effects of AchE inhibitors	
	Reverse muscle paralysis	

Tertiary Amines

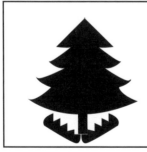 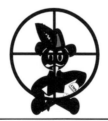 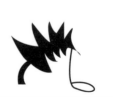

Atropine	**Scopolamine**	**Benztropine**

N	<u>Atropine</u>	<u>A trap</u> in the <u>pines</u> stops the three musketeer cubs from eating fish.
	<u>Scopolamine</u>	Hunter's <u>scope</u> fixed on cubs, so the cubs will <u>be blasted</u> and they won't take the Ace fish from their mother Nicky.
	<u>Benztropine</u>	<u>Bent pine trap</u> snares the cubs and keeps them from getting the fish from Nicky the bear.

mech	Muscarinic cholinergic antagonism	They all keep the cubs from taking fish from their mother.
Dist	Scopolamine ⇒ better entry into CNS than atropine, although atropine does this too	The hunter can get into the University, because he is smarter than a tree.
Tox	Drowsiness and euphoria	The scope makes the cubs go to sleep.
Rt	Scopolamine ⇒ transdermal and PO	

Uses	Atropine:
	    Counteracts all effects (including CNS) of AchE inhibitor poisoning except nicotinic effects
	    Bronchodilation in people with chronic obstructive pulmonary disease (COPD)
	    In general anesthesia to reverse the effects of parasympathomimetic agents
	    Decrease secretions in bronchoscopy
	    To speed up bradycardia
	    Prevent spasm in GU and biliary tract
		¢: From mechanism of action

	Scopolamine ⇒ motion sickness	They won't move because they will be blasted; therefore, it prevents motion sickness.
	Benztropine ⇒ Parkinson's disease	

Tertiary Amines Used Only in Ophthalmology

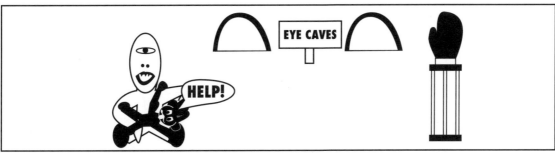

	Cyclopentolate	Tropicamide
N	Cyclopentolate Tropicamide	The cyclops who eats cubs Trophy used to pick his eye.
mech	Muscarinic cholinergic antagonism	The cyclops eats the cubs and keeps them from taking fish from Nicky the bear and playing with the pin. The cubs would rather play with the trophy than take fish from Nicky the bear.
Rt	Intraophthalmic	They are both near the eye cave in the picture.
Uses	Mydriasis	The cubs are wide-eyed and watching for the cyclops and the trophy.

Quaternary Amines Used for Their Antimuscarinic Effects

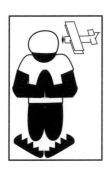

	Ipratropium	**I Pray to Trap 'em**
mech	Muscarinic cholinergic antagonism	I pray to trap the three musketeer cubs and keep them from taking fish from Nicky.
	Because ipratropium is inhaled and not well absorbed, the main action is in the lungs.	I pray to trap them, mainly at the airport.
Dist	Poorly absorbed from lungs	I pray for this only at the airport.

Rt	Inhalation	I <u>fly</u> in to the lake in my floating private plane.
Uses	↓ bronchial secretions and inhibit parasympathetic-mediated bronchoconstriction in chronic obstructive pulmonary disease (COPD) and asthma	I pray hard enough that the rain at the airport stops and the tunnels to the airport open for me ⇒ there is more room for things to fly into the airport.

Propantheline

	Propantheline	**Prowling Panther**
mech	Muscarinic cholinergic antagonism Because propantheline is taken PO and not well absorbed, the main action is in the GI tract.	Eats the cubs if they go to the beach ¢
Dist	Poorly absorbed from GI tract	The panther stays at the beach.
Uses	GI motility or acid secretion	The panther prowls on the beach and prevents the cubs from going down to the beach to release the acid.

Quaternary Amine Used for Ganglionic Blockade

	Trimethaphan	**The Three Mets Fans**
mech	Higher activity at ganglionic blockade	The three Mets fans stop Nick the bear from fishing.
	In the normal state, there is a balance between the PNS and the SNS, blockade of the ganglia → blockade of the predominating system. Therefore, this usually → shift to SNS domination of the organ.	¢
Tox	Anticholinergic and antisympathetic side effects	¢: It blocks the ganglion.
Rt	IV only	
Uses	Only in hypertensive emergencies	Only in horrible traffic, would anyone want to go to a Mets game.

Neuromuscular Junction Blockers—NM Junction Gym

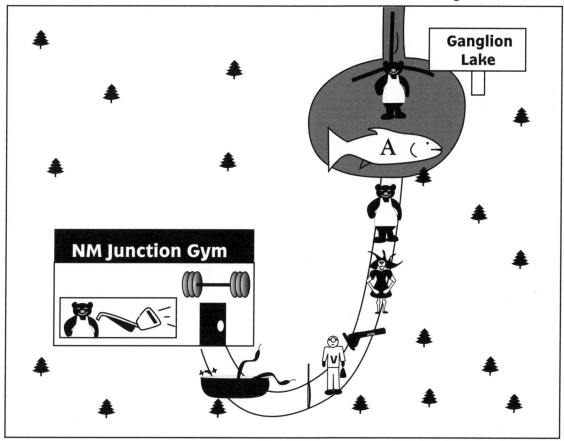

Neuromuscular Junction Physiology and Picture Key

Postsynaptic nerves from the corticospinal tract synapse with skeletal muscle at the neuromuscular junction, using acetylcholine as a neurotransmitter. The skeletal muscle can be viewed as a target organ and as such, we would expect the cholinergic receptors to be muscarinic. It is important to note, however, that this is not the case, as the neuromuscular junction is the only **target organ** that has **nicotinic** cholinergic receptors.

Keeping with the scheme used for the PNS, this picture takes us to the NM Junction Gym, where Nicky works out* after she eats fish at Ganglion Lake. Because the drugs in this chapter cause neuromuscular junction blockade and therein paralysis of the muscle, these drugs interfere with Nicky's workout.

Neuromuscular junction (NMJ)	NM Junction Gym where Nicky works out
Action potential	Nicky goes to the gym after she catches fish at Ganglion Lake.
Cholinergic receptor	The door to the gym. Entrance fee is one Ace fish.
Muscular contraction	After Nicky gets inside → she works out. The work she does is the contraction of the muscle.

---

*If this were a muscarinic cholinergic receptor, the three musketeer cubs would be seen working out.

NMJ Blockers in General

N   Competitive antagonists at cholinergic receptors of NMJ:

           d-Tubocurare
           Pancuronium
           Vecuronium
           Atracurium
           Gallamine

      Depolarizing blockers at NMJ cholinergic receptors:
           Succinylcholine

mech   Quaternary amines paralyze limbs before respiratory muscles

Dist   Not into CNS and thereby do not affect the nicotinic receptors

$t_{1/2}$ Short duration of action

Rt   IV only

Uses   Adjuvant in surgery to obtain paralysis of skeletal muscle → better muscle relaxation to facilitate the surgery at a lower depth of anesthesia
      Facilitate intubation
      Prevent trauma in electroshock therapy

Curfews in combination with things blocking the door to the gym prevent Nicky from entering:
      Tub that blocks the entry to the gym
      A pan that blocks her entry
      Veterinarian—all animals are afraid of vets
      Atra razor that blocks her entry
      A mean gal at the door ⇒ won't let Nicky in.
Things that allow too many Nickys into the gym and thereby make her workout difficult:
A vacuum that sucks Nickys into the gym

¢: They are all quaternary amines.

The blockers are not big things in front of the door, so they can't keep Nicky out for long.

¢: Anytime muscular paralysis may be desired

Competitive Antagonists in General: Things That Keep Nicky Out of the Gym

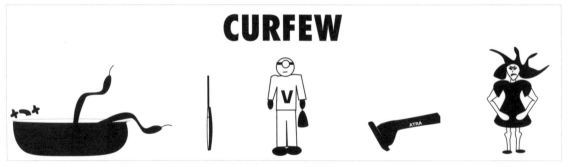

| d-Tubocurare | Pancuronium | Vecuronium | Atracurium | Gallamine |

N   Have -cur- in their name:

           d-Tubocurare
           Pancuronium
           Vecuronium
           Atracurium
           Gallamine

mech   Quaternary amines

      Bind nicotinic cholinergic receptor at the NMJ end-plate → prevents acetylcholine from binding and activating the receptor → paralysis of the muscle

Curfews in combination with things blocking the door to the gym prevent Nicky from entering:
      Tub that blocks the entry to the gym
      Pan that blocks Nicky's entry
      Veterinarian—all animals are afraid of vets
      Atra razor
A mean gal at the door ⇒ won't let Nicky in.
¢: Quaternary amines have good penetration into NMJ.

Block the door to the gym →
      prevent Nicky from entering →
      Nicky can't work out

Dist	Concentrated at NMJ	
Met	Pancuronium and gallamine by kidney	The mean gal carries the pan with her to the shower.
	Vecuronium by liver	The vet is a criminal and is thrown in jail.
	Atracurium by plasma esterases and spontaneous degradation	Atra razors naturally wear out.
Tox	Hypotension ⇒ secondary to direct release of histamine and ganglionic blockade	They can all let hissing snakes out onto the roads, as well as keep Nicky from catching fish at the lake.
	Pancuronium → little to no release of histamine	
Rt	IV	
Uses	d-Tubocurare is seldom used secondary to extensive release of histamine and ganglionic blockade.	The tub has hissing snakes that it carries around and releases as it likes.
R_x/R_x	Some antibiotics can → decreased calcium at the NMJ → decreased release of Ach onto the end plate → enhanced effect of antagonist	
	Cholinesterase inhibitors → reversal of paralysis	

Depolarizing Blockade Paralysis

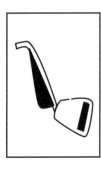

Succinylcholine

The Vacuum That Sucks

N	Succinylcholine	The vacuum that sucks Nicky into the gym.
mech	Binds receptor and activates it → burst of action potentials → muscle fasciculations	The vacuum sucks Nicky into the gym, and they work out until there is no longer space for them to work out.
	Remains bound until it inactivates the Na^+ carrying mechanisms in the end-plate → paralysis	
Met	Plasma cholinesterase	
$t_{1/2}$	Duration of action is very short.	
Tox	Muscle soreness secondary to muscle fasciculations.	So many Nickys that they get sore from being cramped.
	Releases histamine in large doses	If used a lot, it may suck the hissing snakes out of the tub.
R_x/R_x	Paralyzing effect is enhanced with fluorinated anesthetics.	

Sympathetic Nervous System

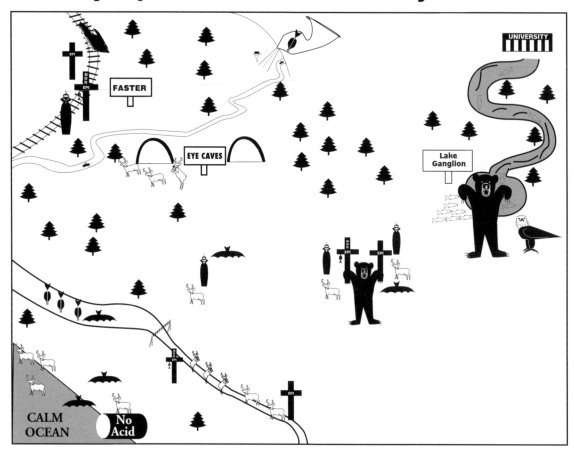

Picture Key

The picture for the sympathetic nervous system lies within the Phunny Pharm Phorest, which depicts the ANS. The SNS picture, however, focuses only on the part of the phorest in which Nick the grizzly bear is found and ignores Nicky, who was the center of attention in the PNS. To review:

In the Body

Binding of <u>acetylcholine</u> to the nicotinic <u>receptor</u> at the <u>ganglion</u>

<u>Postganglionic nerve</u>

<u>Epinephrine (Epi)</u>

<u>Norepinephrine (Norepi)</u>

Adrenergic receptor (i.e., stimulated by Norepi and Epi)
  α_1 and α_2
  β_1

  β_2

In the Phunny Pharm

<u>Nick the grizzly bear</u> catches a <u>fish</u> from the <u>lake</u>.

Nick the grizzly bear's <u>long path</u> after he eats the fish

The cross with <u>Epi</u> on it that Nick uses to chase the animals

The cross with <u>Nor</u> and <u>Epi</u> written on it that Nick uses to chase the animals

<u>Animals</u> who Nick the grizzly bear scares:
  Antelope
  <u>Vampires</u>, which come from bats. Vampires also have <u>one</u> wing (i.e., a cape).
  <u>Bats</u> who have <u>two</u> wings

Binding of <u>norepinephrine</u> to <u>receptor</u> at the <u>target organ</u>	<u>Nick the grizzly bear</u> scares an <u>antelope or a bat</u> with the <u>norepi cross</u>.
Target organ effects of sympathetic nerve stimulation	Things the <u>antelope, vampires, and the bats</u> do after they are scared by Nick

More Picture Keys

The actions of the SNS can be remembered by visualizing the antelope and the bats after they are scared by Nick the grizzly. As they try to get away from Nick, their actions represent the actions at the target organs seen with stimulation of sympathetics and with drugs that mimic the action of norepinephrine. In this, the actions of the antelope and bats can be organized by the long-used cliché, that sympathetics cause a "fight or flight" response.

SNS (3 S's + . . .) (responsible receptor)		**In the Phunny Pharm**
Eyes	My<u>d</u>riasis (<u>d</u>ilate*) (α_1)	Nick scares the antelope out of the eye cave. The antelope <u>make the opening larger</u> as they try to escape out the door. Their <u>eyes are wide</u> with fear.
	Distant vision	Antelope must <u>see long distances</u> to escape predators.
GI tract	Decrease motility (α and β)	After the <u>antelopes</u> and <u>bats</u> are scared, they go to the ocean, drink some water, and make the <u>water calm down</u>.
	Inhibits secretion (α)	The <u>antelope</u> stop acid release into the ocean.
	Inhibits insulin release (α_2)	The <u>antelope</u> decrease sugar in the Phunny Pharm.
	Contraction of sphincters (<u>sphincter</u>) Relaxation of gall bladder	So scared their sphincters are tight
Respiratory tract	Dilation of bronchi (β_2)	The flying <u>bats</u> open (i.e., enlarge) the <u>tunnels to the airports.</u>
Heart	Increase chronotropy (β_1)	The vampires make the conductors of the train drive it faster in fear.
	Increase inotropy (β_1)	They also make it stronger.
Genitals	Ejaculation (<u>shoot</u>) (α_1)	<u>Antelopes</u> (skip this one too)
Urinary tract	Retention (<u>stop</u>) (α_1)	The <u>antelopes</u> do not have to wear diapers.
Arterioles	**Constriction (α_1)**	The <u>antelope</u> run across the highway and close it down when they are scared.
	Dilation (slight) (β_2)	The <u>bats</u> increase the room on the roads.
Veins	**Constriction (α)**	The <u>antelope</u> run to the <u>parking lot</u> to hide when they are scared, thereby leaving little room for cars.
	Dilation (β_2)	The <u>bats</u> open up more room in the parking lot.
Sweat glands	**Localized sweat (<u>s</u>weat) (α_1)**	The <u>antelope make certain areas sweat.</u>

---

*It is difficult to remember that mydriasis = dilate. Just remember that mydriasis has a "d" for dilate, whereas meiosis does not.

Autonomic Reflexes That Modulate Actions of Medications

This topic is very important to understand, because it becomes important in many of the actions of sympathetic drugs. As can be seen from the preceding tables, stimulation of α-receptors at vessels → constriction. In contrast, stimulation of β-receptors at the heart → increased chronotropy and inotropy.

Decrease in blood pressure (BP):

"Sensed" by the carotids → reflex stimulation of the **β-receptors** → tachycardia and increased inotropy

Therefore:

Any **decrease in BP without** concomitant **blockade** of β-receptors will → tachycardia and increased inotropy.

¢: When BP drops, the body tries to maintain cardiac output.

Therefore:

¢: Just go through it a couple of times.

Increase in (BP):

"Sensed" by the carotids → reflex stimulation of the **vagus** → parasympathetic stimulation of the heart → decreased heart rate (HR)

Therefore:

Any **increase in BP without** concomitant **stimulation** of β-receptors will → decreased HR

¢: When BP increases, the body tries to maintain cardiac output

Therefore:

¢: Just go through it a couple of times.

Sympathomimetics—Things That Scare Antelope, Vampires, and Bats

The ability to increase the sympathetic response is very important to all animals' survival; without it we would have been dinner a long, long time ago. Although we only occasionally need it to escape from predators, it has become important to manipulate it in medicine. These sympathetic agonists have been life-saving in diseases such as asthma and anaphylaxis, and instrumental in control of other diseases such as hypotension.

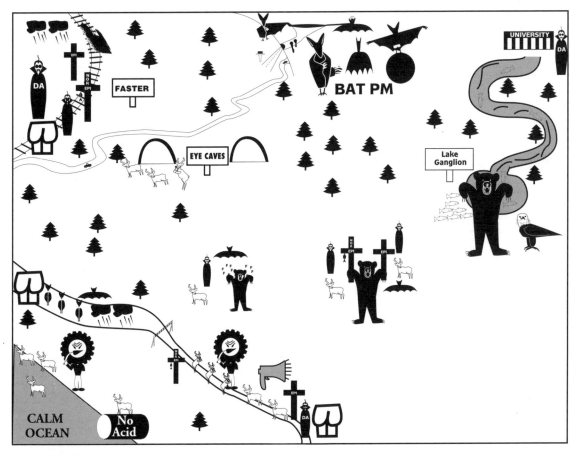

Picture Key

In this picture, we remain in the Phunny Pharm Phorest, but in the SNS, the main focus is on Nick the mean old bear as he scares animals. The actions of the animals when they are scared are the actions that occur with SNS effects. In this, the drugs may be scaring the animals from a distance, up close, or they may be acting like the scared animals.

Indirect-acting agonists	Scare the animals from a long distance; drugs can scare them without physically getting close to them.
Nonspecific-acting agonists	Scare the animals with these drugs; but in the picture, these drugs can be seen with the animals they scare surrounding them, ready to flee.

Specific agonists

These drugs do not rely upon the animals to do something after they scare them. Instead, they carry out the action without worrying about the animals.

Actions can be seen in the SNS Introduction.

Mixed-Acting Agonists

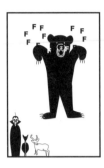

Ephedrine and Mephenteramine

N	Ephedrine and mephenteramine
mech	Stimulates α- and β- receptors and enhances the release of norepinephrine
Rt	PO
Uses	Ephedrine—nasal decongestants and for mydriasis
	Mephenteramine—prevents hypotension induced by spinal anesthesia

The "F" drugs

Nick blows F's out of his nose.
The F's scare antelope, bats, and vampires, and he throws a Norepi cross at the animals.

F's are coming out of his nose, and he can scare the antelope out of the cave.

Indirect-Acting Agonists

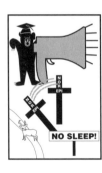

Amphetamine and Methamphetamine

N	Amphetamine and methamphetamine
mech	Induce release of norepinephrine from the presynaptic neurotransmitter vesicles
	→ vasoconstriction → ↑ systolic and diastolic BP
Dist	Well absorbed into CNS
Tox	Decreases appetite, insomnia, nervousness
	Addicting
Rt	PO
Uses	Narcolepsy
	Attention deficit syndrome
	Not useful for weight loss, because tolerance develops to appetite suppression

Amplifiers

Amplifiers that make Nick's mean growl louder and more mean so he can scare the animals from a distance.

Indirectly scares the animals because he only yells at them; he does not physically chase them.

Yells so loud, the antelope run across the road and close it

He has a mortarboard.

When amplifier is around, the antelope and bats are nervous and won't eat.

So loud and mean that antelope and bats do not sleep and it gets the attention of the young animals.

¢: It doesn't work to help decrease appetite for long—Oh well!

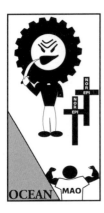

Tyramine

N	Tyramine—Although it is not used as a drug, it has sympathomimetic side effects when ingested in combination with MAO inhibitors.	
mech	Taken up into presynaptic nerve ending → replace norepinephrine from nerve → ↑ norepinephrine in synapses → vasoconstriction and hypertension (HTN)	
Met	Broken down by monoamine oxidase in the gut	
Tox	Can → hypertensive crises	
Rt	PO	
Uses	Not used as a drug, but can be found in cheese, wine, beer . . .	
R_x/R_x	If patient is taking MAO inhibitors, tyramine will make it into the body and → hypertensive crisis.	

Terrible Tire Man

Tire man is walking into the Phunny Pharm from the Ocean, and scaring animals.

He is near the road, so he closes it down.

¢: If there is too much of him
Walking in from ocean

¢: From above

Direct-Acting Agonists

Nonspecific Agonists

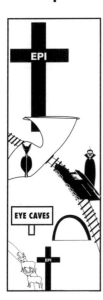

Epinephrine

N	Epinephrine
mech	Stimulates both α- and β-receptors. At low concentrations, β-receptor dominates:
	β_1 → cardiac stimulation → ↑ systolic pressure, and ↑ heart rate
	β_2 → peripheral vasodilation → ↓ total peripheral resistance and diastolic pressure
	At high concentrations, α-receptor dominates: → ↑ vasoconstriction in some vascular beds → ↑ mean arterial BP → vagal reflex → ↓ heart rate
	↑ Coronary blood flow
	Mydriasis
	Bronchial dilation
	Inhibits insulin secretion → ↑ blood glucose
Rt	IV, IM, Inhalation
Uses	Available over the counter as bronchodilator (Primatene Mist)
	Cardiac stimulant and bronchodilator in emergencies.
	Will ↑ BP in anaphylaxis
	With local anesthetics to → local vasoconstriction

Cross with Epi on It

Epi on a cross, which Nick uses to scare vampires, bats, and antelope
Scares both bats and antelope
A couple of small crosses are enough to scare the vampires and bats.
¢: Scares vampires → effects at the heart
¢: Scares bats → effects in vessels

In order to scare the antelope with the cross, Nick must hit the antelope with it. Therefore, he needs a larger cross to do this.

Chases antelope out of eye cave → cave to open more
Can prop open the tunnels to the airport

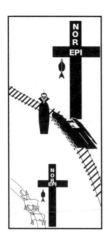

Norepinephrine

N   Norepinephrine is the <u>n</u>eurotrans-
mitter.

mech   Agonist for both α- and β_1 receptors,
but no action at β_2.

    $\beta_1 \rightarrow$ cardiac stimulation $\rightarrow \uparrow$ systolic
pressure, and $\uparrow$ heart rate

    $\alpha \rightarrow \uparrow$ vasoconstriction in some
vascular beds $\rightarrow \uparrow$ mean arterial
BP $\rightarrow$ vagal reflex $\rightarrow \downarrow$ heart rate

    No effect on bronchial dilation
because it has no effect on
β_2-receptors.

NorEpi Cross

A cross with <u>Nor</u> and <u>Epi</u> written on
it, which Nick uses to scare
vampires and antelope.

Antelope and vampires are afraid of
the Norepi cross, but the bats are
not because they cannot see it.*

The Norepi cross scares vampires $\rightarrow$
they scare the train conductor.

The Norepi cross scares antelope $\rightarrow$
they run across the road and shut it
down.

¢: From mechanism

Specific Agonists
α_1-Agonists

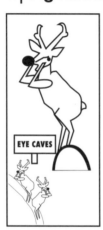

EYE CAVES

Phenylephrine

mech α_1 stimulation $\rightarrow$ vasoconstriction
$\rightarrow \uparrow$ peripheral vascular
resistance $\rightarrow \uparrow$ BP

    Vagal reflex with $\uparrow$ BP $\rightarrow \downarrow$ HR

Met   Not metabolized by catechol-O-
methyltransferase (COMT)

Uses   Nasal decongestant

    Hypotension when vasoconstriction
is desired, as in spinal anesthesia
or sepsis

    Mydriasis

    Vagal reflex can be used to treat
paroxysmal atrial tachycardia.

Funny Little Frightened Antelope

The antelope sets up a road block.

¢: BP increases without β stimulation.

He has a big nose.

He runs out of cave with other antelope.

β-Nonselective Agonists

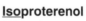
MAO

Isoproterenol

N   Isoproterenol

mech   Stimulate β_1- and β_2-receptors only:

    Iso means equal or alike[†], therefore,
these two work on β_1 and β_2
equally, although isoetharine is
slightly more selective for β_2.

    Stimulation of β_1-receptors $\rightarrow \uparrow$ HR,
inotropy, $\uparrow$ CO.

    Stimulation of β_2-receptors $\rightarrow$ smooth
muscle relaxation $\rightarrow$ bronchodilation
and vasodilation $\rightarrow \downarrow$ peripheral
vascular resistance $\rightarrow \downarrow$ BP

    Get no reflex vagal response
secondary to no α-receptor stimulation

    Decrease vascular permeability

Dist   Mainly remain in lungs when
delivered by aerosol, but systemic
absorption and nonselectivity allow
for side effects

Ice Storm

The ice storm that scares vampires
and bats

Nick the grizzly uses the ice storm to
scare both the vampires and the bats.

¢

¢

¢

Bats do things to the tunnels that $\rightarrow$
them to remain open.

¢: Does not scare antelope

Are bats when they fly into the
tunnels, but if they get into
the blood then they become
vampires and cause side effects

---

*Rem: Bats cannot see.

[†]Barnhart, CL: The World Book Encyclopedia. Chicago, Field Enterprises Educational Corporation, 1965, p. 1044.

$t_{1/2}$	Short	Bats fly very fast.
Met	MAO and chatecol-O-methyltransferase (COMT)	
Tox	Mostly due to activation of β_1-receptors:	Even though they are just bats, they all can change to vampires when they get into the blood.
	Tachycardia	The vampire makes the heart train run faster in fear.
	Tremor	Vampires make everybody tremor with fear.
Rt	<u>Aerosol,</u> not PO	Ice storms <u>fly</u>.
Uses	Used less often than β_2-selective	¢: They are nonselective and have more side effects.

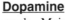

Dopamine

Dopey <u>Dean</u>, the <u>Mean</u> Vampire

mech	Mainly acts as a CNS neurotransmitter, especially in the extrapyramidal system $\Rightarrow$ the "grease" for voluntary muscle movements	He is at the University.
	Precursor of norepinephrine and epinephrine	Scares other vampires into making the train stronger.
	Low doses $\rightarrow$ stimulation of dopaminergic receptors in renal arteries $\rightarrow$ vasodilation	Scares cowboys to speed up their drive to the Phunny Pharm shower
	Higher doses $\rightarrow$ β_1-receptor-agonism $\rightarrow$ increased cardiac contractility	
	Also $\rightarrow$ direct release of norepinephrine	
	Higher doses $\rightarrow$ α_1-receptor agonism $\rightarrow$ vasoconstriction	At high doses, he scares antelope into closing roads.
Uses	Diuresis in CHF	¢: From mechanism
	Hypotension	

β1-Agonists

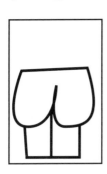

Dobutamine

Dracula's <u>Butt</u> Is <u>a Mean</u> One

mech	β_1-receptor agonist $\rightarrow$ increased cAMP $\rightarrow$ increased Ca entry during contraction $\rightarrow$ increased contractility	Dracula's mean butt scares the vampires to camp out. These vampires make the cows work harder $\rightarrow$ stronger Phunny Pharm Train.
	Also agonist for α and β_2 but $\rightarrow$ no change in peripheral vascular resistance	¢: The effects balance each other out since $\alpha \rightarrow$ vasoconstriction, and $\beta_2 \rightarrow$ vasodilation
$t_{1/2}$	Very short	
Tox	Tachycardia and arrhythmias	¢: From mechanism
Rt	IV only	
Uses	Increase inotropy in CHF	

β₂-Selective Agonists in General

β_2-Selective Agonists in General

BAT PM

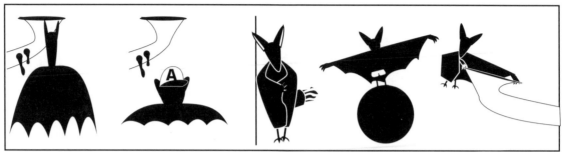

Bitolterol	Albuterol	Terbutaline	Pirbuterol	Metaproterenol

N — All have -ter- in their name and first letters make BAT PM:
- Bitolterol
- Albuterol
- Terbutaline

- Pirbuterol
- Metaproterenol

They cause terror; and bats come out in the PM:

The tall bat bit the wall.

Al the bat bit the wall.

Fast bat ⇒ turbo bat. He leans against the tube wall → enlarge. Turbo bat + lean.

The performing bat, whose butt hit the wall.

The bat who is a pro at tearing the wall.

Tox — Limited 2° to limited systemic absorption and selectivity.

At higher doses, can get absorption

Tremor

Rt — Aerosol-inhaled

Uses — **Symptomatic** relief from asthma

Exercise-induced asthma prophylaxis

Terbutaline and metaproterenol may be used to stop premature labor.

The bats that fly in the PM prefer not to change into vampires.

When there are too many bats, they will get into the blood and change into vampires.

Can shake from fear of these bats

Bats can fly.

¢: From mechanism of action

Sympatholytics—Things That Control Antelope, Vampires, and Bats

A problem with this set of drugs lies in the mechanisms by which many of the sympatholytics act. The α_1-, β_1-, and β_2-receptor direct blockade is relatively straightforward, in that the drug binds the receptor and thereby prevents activation by norepinephrine. The drugs that are not so straightforward are those that act by "indirect mechanisms" and those that stimulate α_2-receptors and actually cause a decrease in sympathetic tone throughout the body.

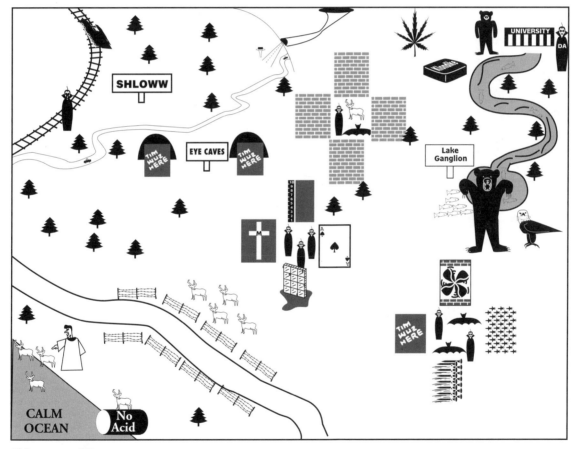

Picture Key

In this picture, we remain in the SNS part of the Phunny Pharm Phorest, where the main focus is upon Nick the mean old bear as he scares animals. Because this is the sympatho**lytics,** we now direct our attention to controlling Nick and to controlling the animals after Nick has scared them. By doing either of these, the animals cannot carry out the actions of the SNS. The drugs that control Nick the bear are those that act by indirect mechanisms, whereas the drugs that control the animals are those that block receptors directly.

Norepinephrine release onto target organ
Norepinephrine binding to receptor
  and causing an action

Nick scaring an animal
The action of the various animals
  after Nick has scared them

Indirect-acting antagonists

Control Nick by making him less scary or by getting him to relax so he will not scare the animals.

Direct-acting antagonists:
  α_1-receptor antagonist
  β_1-receptor antagonist
  β_2-receptor antagonist

Things that control the animals
  Things that control the scared antelope
  Things that control the scared vampires
  Things that control the scared bats

Indirect-Acting Antagonists in General

N   Alpha methyldopa   False messy dope
       Reserpine   Nick becomes reserved.
mech   Indirect-acting antagonists of the sympathetic   These interfere with Nick's ability to scare
       nervous system act by interfering with the   animals.
       normal handling of catecholamines.
       Inhibit norepinephrine synthesis ↑
       norepinephrine's metabolism by blocking
       its movement into neurotransmitter vesicles

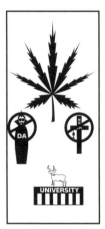

Alpha-methyldopa

mech   Metabolized to "false-transmitters" ⇒
       alpha-methyldopamine and alpha
       methylnorepinephrine (also a potent
       α_2-agonist) → displacement and
       depletion of dopamine and
       norepinephrine from nerves within
       the CNS → decreased outflow of
       sympathetics from the CNS → ↓ BP
       The false messy dope is at the
       University in the picture.
Tox   Sedation, depression, impotence,
       Coombs'-positive hemolytic anemia,
       and hepatitis
Rt   IV and PO
Uses   Hypertensive emergencies
       HTN in pregnancy

False Messy Dope

False messy dope messes up Nick so
that he is not as scary.

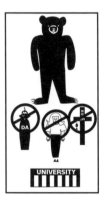

Reserpine

mech   Depletes CNS of norepinephrine,
       dopamine, and serotonin

$t_{1/2}$ 7-day duration of action
Tox   ↓ CNS amines → severe depression
       → suicide
       Sedation, nasal stuffiness, and peptic
       ulcer disease
Rt   IV and PO
Uses   HTN

Nick Becomes Reserved

When Nick becomes reserved, he no
longer wants to scare the animals.
Reserved Nick is at the University
in the picture.

¢: By mechanism of action
   Lowers BP

α_2-Agonists

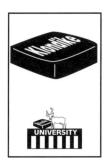

	Clonidine	**Klondike Ice Cream Bars**
mech	α_2 stimulation → ↓ sympathetic outflow from CNS → ↓ peripheral vascular resistance → ↓BP	Antelope eat the Klondike ice cream bars at the University → keeps them from leaving the University.
Dist	Into CNS	Klondike bars are in the University.
Met	May get rebound hypertension when discontinued	Klondike bars can be addicting, such that when they are taken away → ↑ in BP.
Tox	Dry mouth, sedation, and withdrawal	Can withdraw from Klondikes if you quit
Rt	PO and transdermal	Eat Klondike bars.
Uses	HTN	¢: From mechanism of action

Direct-Acting Antagonists

Mixed Antagonists

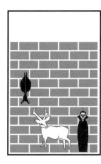

	Labetalol	**Labile Wall**
N	Labetalol, because it ends in -lol, blocks β.	A labile wall that doesn't care which animals it keeps within it.
mech	α_1-, β_1-, and β_2-adrenergic blockers	Labile wall controls antelope, vampires, and bats.
Rt	PO or IV	
Uses	HTN	
	Clonidine withdrawal	

Nonspecific α-Antagonists

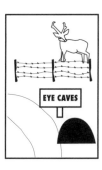

	Phentolamine and Phenoxybenzamine	**Fences That Control Antelope**
mech	α_1- and α_2-adrenergic blockers: Phentolamine is a competitive α-antagonist Phenoxybenzamine is a noncompetitive α-antagonist → inhibition of vasoconstriction of sympathomimetics → ↓ BP ↓ in BP → reflex tachycardia because the β-receptors are not blocked	These fences control the antelope and do not let them get scared by Nick.* They do this at the University and elsewhere. Control the antelope and keep them from blocking the road. ¢
Tox	Postural hypotension and reflex tachycardia	¢: From mechanism of action
	Miosis	Keep antelope from running out of eye cave and making the opening larger
	Nasal stuffiness	
Uses	HTN emergencies secondary to pheochromocytosis	
	Vascular disease ⇒ Raynaud's	

---

*For you who do not know, antelope have a very hard time getting through fences, whereas deer and elk have no trouble at all.

α_1-Antagonists

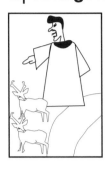

Prazosin and Terazosin

mech Inhibition of α_1-receptors prevents constriction of arterioles → ↓ blood pressure.

Tox First dose must be given slowly, because hypotension can result with the first dose.

Uses HTN
Benign prostatic hypertrophy (BPH)

Preys Upon and Terrorizes Antelope Sinners

He controls the antelope sinners and prevents them from making road blocks.

¢: From mechanism of action

β-Adrenergic Blockers in General

N   End in -olol
Nonselective β-antagonists:
Propranolol
Nadolol
Timolol
Pindolol
β_1-specific antagonists:
Metoprolol
Atenolol
Acebutolol
Esmolol

mech β-blockade inhibits reflex tachycardia seen with other antihypertensives.
Inhibits sympathetic tone on heart → negative inotropy and negative chronotropy

↓ renin release

Tox β-blockade effects → congestive heart failure,* brochospasm in asthmatics (related mainly to β_2-crossreactivity), AV block, diabetes

Uses HTN
Angina
Arrhythmias
Prevention of MI following previous MI
Used carefully in CHF

All symbolized by a wall:
Control vampires and bats:
Propeller wall
Wall made of nails
Tim's wall
Pin wall
Walls that control only vampires:
Methodist church wall
A ten-foot-high wall
Ace wall
Eskimo wall

β_1-receptors are blocked, therefore, β_1-receptors cannot be used to correct the fall in BP.

¢: These are the actions of β-receptor blockade. In the picture, they slow down the train by keeping the vampires from scaring the conductor.

¢: From mechanism of action.

¢: This is one of their main effects.

They slow down the conductor.

β1- and β2-Nonselective Adrenergic Blockers in General

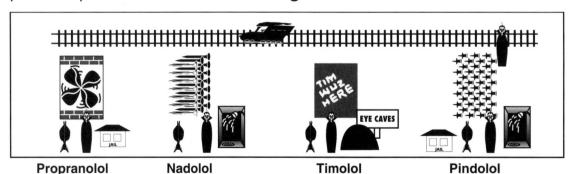

| Propranolol | Nadolol | Timolol | Pindolol |

*Although β-blockers can cause CHF, they are beginning to be used in select cases to treat CHF by "upregulating" adrenergic receptors.

N	Propranolol	Propeller wall	
	Nadolol	Wall made of nails	
	Timolol	Tim's wall	
	Pindolol	Pin wall	
mech	Inhibits sympathetic stimulation of the heart (essentially rests the heart)	These walls keep the vampires and bats from scaring the conductor of the train.	
	Heart rate ↓ ⇒ allows for longer diastole and therefore longer time for coronary blood to flow.	Keeps the vampires from speeding up the train	
	↓ inotropy		
	→ bronchoconstriction	Keeps the bats from opening the tubes to the airport	
	Pindolol ⇒ may also have some intrinsic sympathomimetic effects → less depression of HR and CO	The pins on the wall may snag the vampires' wings and scare them.	
Dist	Nadolol ⇒ does not enter the CNS	The nail wall is not at the University.	
Met	Propranolol ⇒ hepatic	A jail is next to the propeller wall.	
	Nadolol ⇒ renal	A shower is next to the nail wall.	
	Pindolol ⇒ hepatic and renal	A shower and jail are next to the pin wall.	
$t_{1/2}$	Nadolol ⇒ longer acting ⇒ may be give once a day	The nail wall controls the vampires and bats for longer periods of time, as they are afraid of the sharp points of the nails.	
Tox	Relatively contraindicated in asthmatics	¢: Can cause bronchoconstriction when it blocks the bronchodilatory effects of β_2-receptor stimulation.	
	Relatively contraindicated in diabetes ⇒ will ↑ blood glucose and will inhibit tachycardia if patient becomes hypoglycemic	Walls decrease the glucose in the Phunny Pharm.	
	Depression	¢: These are effects of β-blockade.	
	Impotence		
Rt	PO		
	Timolol ⇒ intraophthalmic		
Uses	Propranolol ⇒ tremor and stage fright (i.e., performance anxiety)	The propeller wall keeps the vampires and bats from making the streets of the Phunny Pharm tremble with fear.	
	Timolol ⇒ open-angle glaucoma (↓ aqueous humor formation)		

β1-Specific Antagonists

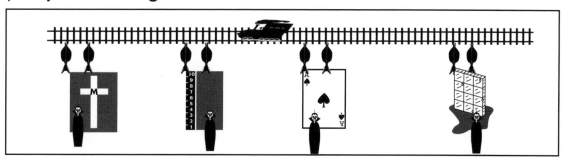

	Metoprolol	Atenolol	Acebutolol	Esmolol

N	The first letters spell "AAME"	These walls have a better "AIM" at the β_1.	
	Atenolol	A ten-foot-high wall keeps the vampires in but the bats can fly right over.	

	<u>Acebuto</u>lol	<u>Ace wall</u> stops the vampire but not the bat.
	<u>Meto</u>pro<u>lol</u>	<u>Metho</u>dist church <u>wall</u>, which definitely scares the vampire
	<u>Es</u>molol	<u>Eskimo wall</u> freezes the vampires, but not the bats.
mech	Blocks β_1 selectively $\Rightarrow$ essentially, no effect on lungs and glucose metabolism; therefore, can be used in asthmatics and diabetics **more** safely	These only stop the vampires.
	<u>Acebuto</u>lol $\Rightarrow$ has some sympathomimetic activity in addition to its β_1-blockade	
Met	Metoprolol $\Rightarrow$ hepatic	
	Atenolol $\Rightarrow$ renal	
$t_{1/2}$	Esmolol is a very short acting β-blocker.	The Eskimo ice wall melts rapidly.
	Atenolol $\Rightarrow$ longer $t_{1/2}$	
Tox	Smaller risk of asthma exacerbation and worsened control of diabetes	¢: Because of selective β_1-blockade.

Central Nervous System—The Phunny Pharm University

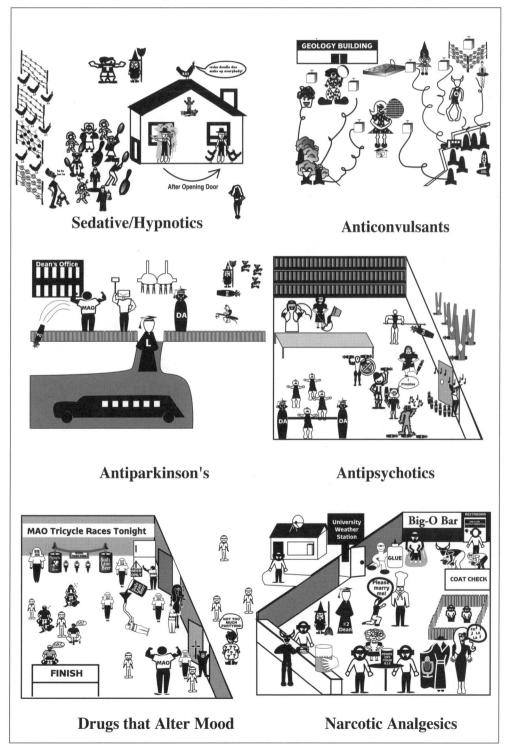

Sedatives and Hypnotics—The University Pharm

A **sedative** reduces anxiety and excitement, whereas a **hypnotic** induces sleep. Owing to their similar actions, the sedative/hypnotics are easy to group into a single category. They have long been used as tranquilizers, sleeping pills, and anxiolytics, but also have uses as anesthetics and anticonvulsants. This chapter introduces the most widely used sedative/hypnotics, benzodiazepines and barbiturates. Be sure to remember, however, that you will find them in other chapters.

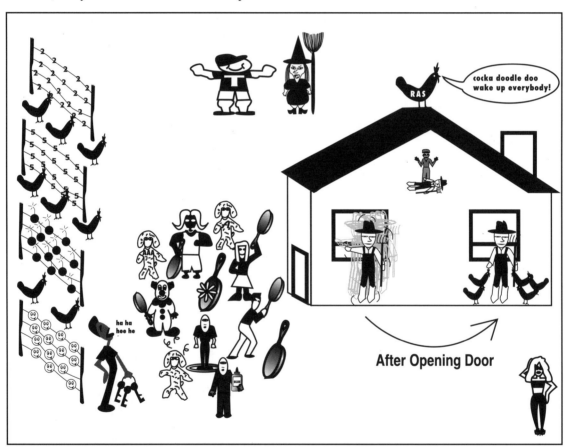

Picture Key

This chapter takes us to the agricultural department of the Phunny Pharm University, where we find the the University Pharm (i.e., Farm). There is much anxiety and confusion at this farm. The farmer represents the patient in this picture, and his anxiety is the problem that is treated by the medications in this chapter. Fortunately, there are some chickens who have not lost their heads, and they help to restore some calm and serenity to the farmer. It is **not** important to understand **how** the chickens combat the anxiety, only that the more chickens that surround the farmer, the less the anxiety.

The sedative/hypnotics that are depicted in this chapter are the benzodiazepines and barbiturates. They are represented by things that increase the number of chickens around the farmer. There is a difference in the way barbiturates and benzodiazepines get this done. You could call it a difference in approach. The benzodiazepines are much gentler in doing their duty, whereas the barbiturates can sometimes be as rough as "barbed wire."

Chloride	Chickens
Nerve cells in the brain	The farm house at the University Farm
Anxiety	Anxiety felt by the farmer
Reticular activating system ≅ keeps the brain awake	A rooster in the farm house that keeps the farmer awake
Sedation	The rooster is distracted so that he cannot keep the farmer awake → the farmer falls asleep.
GABA receptor	A doorkeeper at the farm house who allows chickens into the house when GABA is around.
Stimulation of GABA receptors → influx of Cl into the nerve → increased inhibition of neurons	GABA → the doorkeeper allows chickens to come into the farm house → calms the farmer in the house.
Benzodiazapines	Things that convince the door keeper to let chickens into the farm house
Barbiturates	Barbed wire fences that help direct chickens into the farm house

Benzodiazepines In General

The benzodiazepines have replaced the barbiturates as the sedative/hypnotics of choice. Their safer nature and lower abuse potential have allowed them to come into widespread use as sedative/hypnotics, anticonvulsants, and antianxiety agents. The main feature that separates the individual benzodiazepines is their pharmacokinetics, and this will guide you in choosing the appropriate benzodiazepine.

N	Short-acting benzodiazepines: end in -lam or -pam and begin with L,O,T M, and A		
		Oxazepam	An ox uses a pan against the doorkeeper
		Alprazolam	Alpo lamb is so soft that the doorkeeper can't resist.
		Lorazepam	Lora raises a pan at the doorkeeper.
		Triazolam	A lamb with three A's convinces the doorkeeper.
		Temazepam	Tim with a pan, uses it against the doorkeeper.
		Midazolam	My dazed lamb convinces the doorkeeper.
	Long-acting benzodiazepines: begin with C, D, or F		
		Diazepam	Daisies in a pan are pretty → relax the doorman.
		Clonazepam	Clown with a pan, which he uses to hit the doorman.
		Clorazepate	Chlor, the cyclops on a plate, gets the doorman.
		Chlordiazepoxide	Chlor, the cyclops epoxide ⇒ glues the doorman
		Flurazepam	A pan that floors the doorman
mech	Bind to the benzodiazepine site on the GABA receptor → Cl influx → inhibition of the postsynaptic nerve		They all make the doorkeeper let the chickens into the farm house → calm the farmer down.
Dist	Highly protein bound		
Met	All are metabolized mainly by the liver.		All may go to jail.
Tox	Sedation (in some cases, this is a desired clinical effect)		The chickens (especially the hens) distract the rooster, who is supposed to keep the farmer awake.
	Ataxia		

Alcoholics may experience euphoria ⇒ they
    have ↑ abuse potential.

Fetal malformations with first trimester use

Rare fatal overdose

Rt   All can be used PO.

Uses   Sedation ≡ hypnosis; therefore,   ¢: They calm the farmer, may make him
        can treat insomnia   tired, and even put him to sleep.
        Seizure prevention and treatment: They also prevent earthquakes.
          Alcohol withdrawal
          Anticonvulsant
          Status epilepticus
        Anesthesia   Can use them to put people to sleep for
                                operations.

        Muscle relaxation   They allow enough chickens into the NM
                                Junction Gym such that no muscles are used.

        Preoperative as an anxiolytic
        Some anxiety disorders

Short-Acting Benzodiazepines

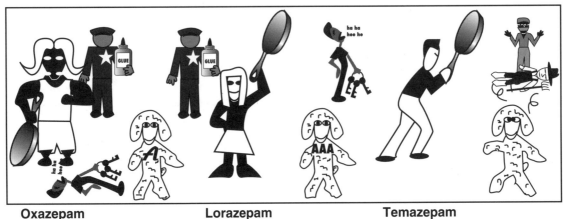

Oxazepam   Lorazepam   Temazepam
      Alprazolam   Triazolam   Midazolam

N   End in -lam or -pam and begin with
        L,O,T, M, and A
          Oxazepam   An ox uses a pan against the doorkeeper
          Alprazolam   Alpo lamb is so soft that the doorkeeper can't
                                  resist.
          Lorazepam   Lora raises a pan at the doorkeeper.
          Triazolam   A lamb with three A's convinces the
                                  doorkeeper.
          Temazepam   Tim with a pan uses it against the doorkeeper.
          Midazolam   My dazed lamb convinces the doorkeeper.

Met   Glucuronidation, mainly by the liver, results   When glue is put on them by the policeman,
        in inactive metabolites.   they cannot get to the doorkeeper.
        Oxazepam, lorazepam, and alprazolam   A policeman imposter can glue the ox, Lora, and
          undergo glucuronidation at hepatic and   the Alpo lamb.
          extra-hepatic sites before urinary
          excretion (i.e., good for liver failure
          patients).
        They all form metabolites that are not active.*
        Temazepam is mainly glucuronidated, but   Tim with a pan is not just glued to the floor.
          may have other active metabolites.

---

*Triazolam, alprazolam, and midazolam form metabolites that are very short-lived, so they can be considered nonactive.

shortest.

one by morning.

nocks out the farmer so the
erate.

tes that are formed during their

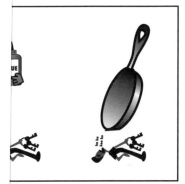

poxide   Flurazepam

are pretty → relax the doorman.
n, which he uses to hit the

ps on a <u>plate</u>, gets the doorman.
ps <u>epoxide</u> ⇒ glues the

the doorman
ps on a plate, has to come off his
e can go to the University

the cyclops on a plate, and Chlor
ide here the Norse pictured

rs the doorman does not
orse.

Diazepam and chlordiazepoxide ⇒ IV and PO
Clorazepate ⇒ PO only

Uses   Diazepam, clorazepate, and chlordiazepoxide
      ⇒ anxiety
Flurazepam ⇒ insomnia, despite the long $t_{1/2}$
Clonazepam ⇒ mainly used for seizures
Chlordiazepoxide ⇒ outpatient alcohol detox

¢: Clorazepate is a prodrug and has to be
activated in the stomach.

Benzodiazepine Antagonist

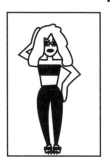

Flumazenil

N	Flumazenil	
mech	Reverses all effects of benzodiazepines	
Met	Liver	
$t_{1/2}$	Short $\Rightarrow$ <1 hr	
Uses	Reverse benzodiazepine overdose	

Amazing Floozy

An <u>amazing floozy</u> who closes the door and chases chickens out of the farm house.

Opposite action of the benzodiazepines

She is thrown in jail for solicitation.

¢

Barbiturates in General

The barbiturates have long been used as sedative/hypnotics; however, because of significant toxicity and problems with dependence and withdrawal, they have been replaced, for the most part, by the much safer benzodiazepines. They continue to be used in anesthesia, as anticonvulsants, and to reduce intracerebroventricular pressure associated with trauma, ischemic brain injury, and neurosurgery.

Barbiturates are classified on the basis of duration of action: ultra-short–acting, short-to-intermediate–acting, and long-acting.

N   Ultra-short–acting barbiturates:

These are both pictured as people and therefore can't affect the doorkeeper as long as the fences can.

Thiopental

<u>Theo pens</u> them <u>all</u> so the chickens will enter the house.

Methohexital

<u>Martha hexes</u> them <u>all,</u> convincing the doorkeeper to allow the chickens into the house.

Short-to-intermediate–acting barbiturates:

Barbed wire that is placed around the chickens to help direct them into the house:

Pentobarbital   Number <u>five</u> barbed wire
Secobarbital   Number <u>second</u> barbed wire
Amobarbital   <u>Ammo</u> (ammunition) barbed wire
Long-acting barbiturates:
Phenobarbital

The <u>phunny</u> <u>barbed</u> wire makes the doorkeeper laugh until he lets the chickens into the house.

mech   At low doses, barbiturates stimulate GABA receptors → increases inhibitory effect of that receptor. This is especially important when it acts on the <u>reticular activating system</u> → resulting in sedative effects.

At first, the barbed wire fences only make the doorkeeper let chickens into the house → The chickens calm the farmer. This is especially important when the chickens distract the <u>rooster</u> who is responsible for keeping the farmer awake → the rooster lets the farmer sleep.

At higher doses, they act by general neuronal membrane perturbation, resulting in hypnotic/anesthetic effects.

The more they are there, however, the rougher they get, because they may directly attack the farmer to calm him down.

Met   Oxidation and dealkylation in liver

The barbed wire fences are thrown in jail when they finish.

Tox   <u>Respiratory</u> depression

Barbed wires stretch across the runways of the <u>Phunny Pharm Airport</u> and prevent planes from landing.

Myo<u>cardial</u> depression leading to severe hypotension

Barbed wires stretch across the tracks of the <u>Phunny Pharm Train.</u>

May precipitate acute attacks of porphyria
Abrupt withdrawal → seizures, delirium, insomnia, tremor, and anorexia

When the barbed wires leave quickly, the farmer isn't ready to be on his own, so he quakes and shakes, can't sleep, and doesn't eat.

Ultra-Short–Acting Barbiturates

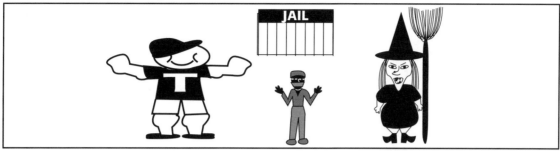

	Thiopental	**Methohexital**
N	Thiopental	Theo pens them all so the chickens will enter the house.
	Methohexital	Martha hexes them all, convincing the doorkeeper to allow the chickens into the house.
Dist	Very large secondary to high lipid solubility	They are both very fat.
Met	Hepatic	They get thrown into jail for kidnapping the chickens.
t$_{1/2}$	Rapid onset of action	They both act very fast because they do not have to build a barbed wire fence before they can work.
Rt	IV	
Uses	Induction of anesthesia by IV	¢: A good use for these because they work so rapidly.
	There is rapid emergence from anesthesia because they redistribute to less vascularized tissues having high fat content.	When they leave, the farmer awakens rapidly.

Short-to-Intermediate–Acting Barbiturates

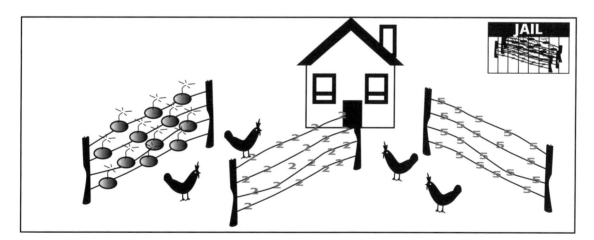

	Amobarbital	**Secobarbital**	**Pentobarbital**
N	Short-to-intermediate–acting barbiturates:		Barbed wire that is placed around the chickens to help direct them into the house.
	All end in -barbital:		They are all tall barbed wire fences:
	Amobarbital		Ammo (ammunition) barbed wire
	Secobarbital		Number second barbed wire
	Pentobarbital		Number five barbed wire

Met	Liver microsomal enzymes	They get thrown in jail when they are through ⇒ they are used to make better jail cells.
Uses	Infrequently used as sedatives because they are very addictive	When they tie up the doorkeeper, they are very abusive, so they are not used much.
	Pentobarbital ⇒ induce coma to terminate status epilepticus	The number five fence is used to stop severe earthquakes.

Long-Acting Barbiturates

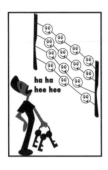

Phenobarbital

N	Phenobarbital	
Met	30% excreted unchanged in urine	
$t_{1/2}$	Long-acting	
Uses	Can be used as an anticonvulsant because of its longer half-life	

Phunny Barbed Wire

The phunny barbed wire makes the doorkeeper laugh until he lets the chickens into the house.

30% of the barbed wire is taken to the shower.

Phunny barbed wire wraps bad guys, which prevents them from detonating explosives and causing earthquakes.*

---

*See the upcoming chapter on anticonvulsants ⇒ explosions at the Phunny Pharm University represent seizures.

Anticonvulsants—Earthquake Prevention

An Introduction to Epilepsy

Epilepsy is a group of chronic CNS disorders characterized by recurrent seizures. A seizure is an abnormal excessive discharge of neurons in the brain that results in motor, sensory, psychological, or behavioral activities. Seizures can be separated into two categories, generalized or focal (partial).

Generalized seizures: Associated with abnormal discharge of the entire cortex with loss of conciousness
Classification:

<u>Tonic–clonic seizures</u> result in sustained tonic contractions, jerking clonic contractions, or alternating contraction/relaxation of the skeletal muscles. The patient may also bite his tongue or be incontinent of urine. They are always followed by a postictal period.

<u>Absence</u> seizures result in loss of conciousness that last only seconds.

Treatment: All anticonvulsants listed in this chapter can be used for generalized seizures, although some are specific for absence seizures.

Partial ≡ focal seizures: Seizures associated with abnormal discharge of only a focal area of cortex
Classification:

<u>Simple seizures</u> result in simple motor, sensory, or special sensory symptoms in only one part of the body. They do not impair consciousness.

<u>Complex seizures</u> impair consciousness and are often preceded by an aura. They result in strange psychological experiences and odd behavior.

<u>Secondarily generalized</u> ⇒ both simple and complex seizures can become generalized.

Treatment: Carbamazepine, valproate, and phenytoin can be used.

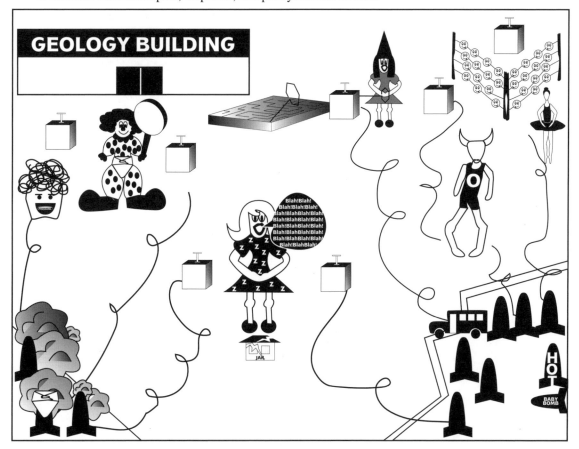

Picture Key

For the anticonvulsants, we travel to the geology building on the University campus. Here, the earthquake preventors conduct their research.

Abnormal firing of a neuron	An explosion detonated by the bad guys
Seizure	Earthquakes caused by explosions:
Generalized	Large earthquakes caused by large explosions
Partial	Small earthquakes caused by small explosions
Absence seizures	Smoke bombs set off by the bad guys that result in an earthquake, but it is more of an inability to do anything for a few seconds; you cannot see.

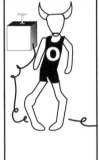

Phenytoin

mech	Stabilizes neuronal membranes ⇒ ↓ sodium and potassium currents → suppress repetitive firing of neurons.	**Steers Who Walk <u>Funny</u>—<u>Toes in</u>** The steer walks funny with his toes in and trips on the wires leading from the detonator to the explosives → prevents detonation ⇒ prevents the earthquake.
Dist	90% protein bound	
Met	Follows zero-order kinetics	He has a zero on his chest.
Tox	Cognitive impairment	He can't think straight.
	Non–dose-related:	With any amount of phenytoin, you may begin to look like a steer ⇒ hairy, coarse facial features, and thick gums.
	Hypertrichosis	
	Coarsening of facial features	
	Gingival hyperplasia	
	Dose-related: nystagmus, ataxia, lethargy, coma	With a lot of phenytoin, you get nystagmus; you walk funny ataxic and are lethargic.
Uses	All seizure types except absence	The steer doesn't care about smoke bombs.

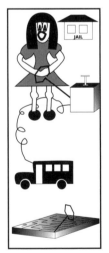

Carbamazepine

N	<u>Carbamazepine</u>	**Throws the <u>Car Bomb Pin</u>** She throws the detonator <u>pin</u> of the <u>car bomb</u> into <u>a maze</u> so the bad guys can not find it.
mech	Carbamazepine and an active metabolite have actions similar to phenytoin.	She can walk funny with her toes in and trip over the wire running from the detonator to the explosives.
Dist	75% protein bound	
Met	Induces its own metabolism in the liver	She is honest. She locks herself in jail after she steals the detonator pin.
Uses	Partial seizures	She prevents both big and small earthquakes.
	Generalized tonic-clonic	
	Mixed	
	Peripheral neuropathy	She can take away pain.
	Rapidly cycling manic-depressive episodes	She also is friends with Letha the MAO Fraternity house mother.*

---

*Rem: Letha represents lithium, the drug of choice for manic depression in most cases; as will be noted in the upcoming chapter on antidepressants.

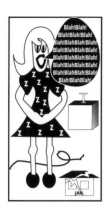

Valproate

mech	Unknown, but may ↑ brain GABA levels	
Dist	90% protein bound	
Tox	Gastric upset	
	Sedation	
	<u>Hepatic</u> toxicity	
	Blood dyscrasias	
	↑ spina bifida in fetuses	
Uses	Absence seizures	
	Mixed seizures	

Val, Pro Earthquake Preventor

Val gets the bad guys to gabbing so they forget to detonate the explosion and therein prevents earthquakes.

She makes waves in the ocean.
She talks so much, she puts the patient to sleep.
Val destroys the <u>jail</u>.
Bad blood between her and the bad guys after she gets them to gabbing
She doesn't like babies.
She hates smoke bombs and does everything within her power to prevent them.
She prevents earthquakes—big and small.

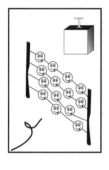

Phenobarbital

mech	Barbiturate—stimulates GABA receptors → influx of chloride into the cell → decreases the excitability of the nerve	
Tox	Non–dose-related:	
	Impaired short-term memory	
	Hyperactivity in children	
	Allergic dermatitis	
	Stevens-Johnson syndrome	
	Dose-related:	
	Sedation	
	Mental dullness	
	<u>Ataxia</u>	
Uses	Generalized tonic–clonic seizures	
	Partial seizures	
	Neonatal seizures	
	Febrile seizures	
R_x/R_x	Induces P450 enzymes ⇒ ↑ metabolism of many drugs such as phenytoin, digoxin, and coumadin	

Phunny Barbed Wire

The phunny barbed wire fence makes the doorkeeper allow chickens into the geology building → the chickens calm the bad guys so they won't detonate the explosive.

The fence is so phunny, it makes kids hyperactive.

The chickens inhibit the rooster,* who is responsible for keeping the people awake.

It's <u>hard to walk</u> with barbed wire wrapped around you.
Prevents both large and small earthquakes by stopping the explosives

Prevents baby bombs from exploding
Prevents hot bombs from exploding

---

*Rem: The rooster represents the reticular activating system (RAS = rooster) as seen in the chapter on sedatives.

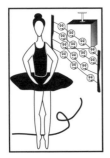

Primidone

mech	Actions similar to phenobarbital
Met	Metabolized to phenobarbital

A Primadonna

The primadonna builds a phunny barbed wire fence.

After she builds the fence, she leaves it up to the phunny barbed wire to prevent the explosions.

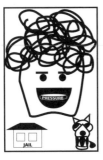

Ethosuximide

mech	Unknown
Dist	Not protein-bound
Met	In liver to inactive metabolites
Tox	Dose-related:
	Gastric distress
	Anorexia
	Drowsiness
	Headache
	Lupus-like syndrome—rarely
Uses	Absence seizures

Ethyl Sucks the Mine

Don't know how, but Ethyl sucked the mine so that it could not explode.

She goes to jail.

A wolf can be seen in the picture with Ethyl.

She is a smoker. She sucks on the smoke bomb so that it will not explode.

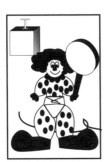

Clonazepam

mech	Benzodiazepine—binds to the benzodiazepine site on the GABA receptor → Cl influx → inhibition of the postsynaptic nerve.
Tox	Tolerance
Uses	Absence seizures when other drugs have not worked

The Clown with a Pan

The clown hits the doorkeeper so that he lets the chickens into the geology building → calms the bad guys so they won't detonate their explosives.

Antiparkinson's—Making the University Run

Introduction to Parkinson's Disease

Parkinson's disease is a disease of motion. Unfortunately, there is no cure for this dreadful disease, whose course is chronic and progressive, but there are treatments that improve the quality of life and perhaps even slow the disease's progression.

Symptoms seem to be due to the loss of dopaminergic neurons in the substantia nigra. If you can think of dopamine produced by these neurons as "grease" for movement, then the loss of these neurons is similar to putting the "brakes" on all voluntary movements. This results in bradykinesia (i.e. slow movements), postural instability, rigidity, tremor, and dementia.

A theory on the loss of neurons in the substantia nigra in Parkinson's disease: MPTP was an attempt to synthesize "street demerol." The unfortunate people who took this drug developed a Parkinsonian-like syndrome. The problem was that the MPTP was metabolized to MPP^+ (a free radical) by the monoamine oxidase system, and the free radical destroyed the dopaminergic nerves of the substantia nigra. Therefore, it is hypothesized that there is an environmental toxin similar to MPTP.

Treatment consists of increasing the amount of dopamine available to the neurons in the substantia nigra. In addition, the balance between the dopaminergic neurons and the cholinergic neurons of the substantia nigra is important in maintaining the grease in movement. Cholinergic neurons keep the normal dopaminergic neurons in check. With the loss of dopaminergic neurons seen in Parkinson's disease, there is an excess cholinergic activity, such that inhibition of cholinergic receptors will result in a pseudo-increase in dopamine.

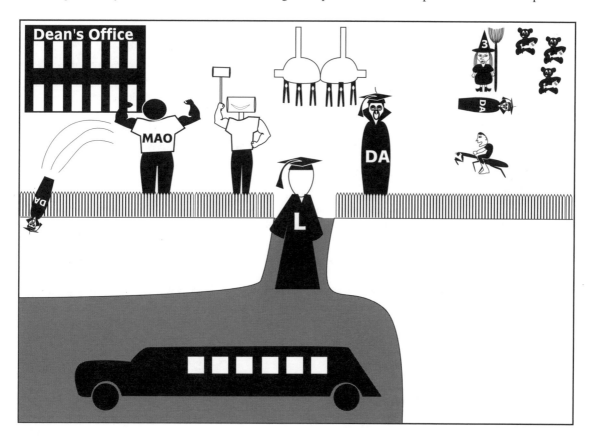

Picture Key

In this chapter, we continue with our tour of the Phunny Pharm University. Here, we look into the internal workings of the administration of the University. The <u>dopey dean</u> is the "grease." He needs to be there so that things operate smoothly. When he's not at the University, the system comes to a screeching halt and we get Parkinson's disease. On the other hand, if he's there too much, the University has excess "grease" and things get a little crazy ⇒ we become schizophrenic.

Dopamine (DA)

"Dopey" dean of the University: He is a vampire that will suck your wallet dry with his tuition ↑.

<u>L</u>-Dopa ⇒ precursor to DA

The dean on his way to the University is a <u>l</u>azy dean.

Dopa-<u>decarboxylase</u>—an enzyme everywhere in the body that turns L-dopa into DA.

Bad guys in the Phunny Pharm that keep the lazy, dopey dean away from the university (take him out of his car)

<u>Substantia</u> nigra

The dean's <u>substantial</u> office

Blood–brain barrier (<u>BBB</u>)

The parking lot <u>boundaries</u> that separate the University from the rest of the body

<u>Monoamine oxidase enzyme system</u>

The <u>bouncer</u> of the <u>Mu Alpha Omega Fraternity house</u> who throws the dean out of the University

Loss of dopaminergic neurons

Damage to the dean's substantial office

Cholinergic neurons

The three musketeer cubs interfere with the dopey dean, such that he can't get his work done.

Anticholinergic

Things that stop the three musketeer cubs and allow the dean to function normally ⇒ allow movement at the University.

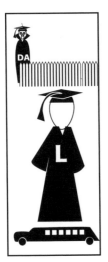

L-Dopa and Carbidopa

N	<u>L</u>-<u>d</u>opa and <u>carbidopa</u>
mech	L-dopa—which is <u>decarboxylated</u> in the brain by <u>dopa-decarboxylase</u> → ↑ dopamine → improved Parkinson's symptoms
	<u>Carbidopa</u>—inhibitor of dopa-decarboxylase. This ↓ the peripheral decarboxylation of L-dopa ⇒ need reduced dosages of L-dopa to get sufficent drug in brain. This also reduces systemic toxicity.
Dist	L-dopa passes readily into CNS.
	Carbidopa does not cross BBB.
Met	Without carbidopa only 1% of L-dopa reaches the brain due to decarboxylation in the periphery
Tox	Nausea
	Hypotension
	Cardiac arrhythmias

Lazy Dean and His Car

The <u>l</u>azy <u>d</u>opey dean on his way to work, who rides in the <u>car</u> of the <u>dopey</u> dean

The lazy dean becomes the dopey dean when he is <u>taken out of his car</u> at the University.

The <u>car of the dean</u> ensures that the dean arrives at the University.

The lazy dean can go into the University.

The car of the dopey dean must remain in the parking lot.

Without the special <u>car</u> of the <u>dopey dean</u>, he never gets to the University.

¢: Too much DA in the periphery → nausea

Does not make ¢, but L-dopa can do it anyway

The lazy dean interferes with the conductor of the train.

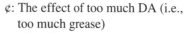

	Involuntary movements	¢: The effect of too much DA (i.e., too much grease)
	Psychiatric disturbances	¢: The effect of too much DA (see antipsychotic chapter)
Rt	PO	

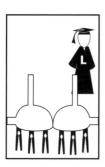

Selegiline

mech	Selective MAO-B inhibitor	
	Inhibitor of dopamine uptake pump	
Tox	Hypomania	
	Psychosis	
	Hypotension	
Rt	PO	
Uses	May slow progression of disease	
	Can use with L-dopa	

The Sledgehammer

Sledgehammer is a member of the Mu Alpha Omega Fraternity who smashes the bouncer when he takes the dopey dean out of the University.

He has a smiley face.
He participates in the party at the library.

Sledgehammer protects the substantial office and makes sure it is around for years to come.
Sledgehammer is a friend of the lazy dean.

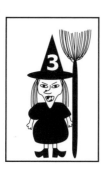

Bromocriptine

mech	Direct dopamine agonist	
$t_{1/2}$	1.5–3 hr	
Tox	Nausea and vomiting	
	Hypotension	
Rt	PO	
Uses	May use with L-dopa	
	Hyperprolactinemia ⇒ release of prolactin is inhibited by dopamine	

A Bra with Mo' Clips

The dean's best supporter.

¢: Too much dopamine makes you throw up.
The bra makes the dean's blood pressure drop.

¢: It is a bra ⇒ helps with gynecomastia associated with the hyperprolactinemia.

Trihexyphenidyl

mech	Anticholinergic ⇒ restores balance between dopaminergic and cholinergic neurons.	
$t_{1/2}$	Long	
Tox	Anticholinergic side effects	
Rt	PO	
Uses	Treats the tremor and rigidity in Parkinson's disease	

The Witch of Three Hexes

The witch puts a hex on the three musketeer cubs and restores the dopey dean to power.
She has a long broom.
The three musketeer cubs can't do anything with three hexes on them.

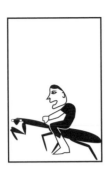

Amantadine

mech	Stimulates release of dopamine— exact mechanism unknown
Tox	Few side effects Possible hallucinations at high doses
Rt	PO
Uses	Early stages of disease

A Cowboy Riding a Mantis

The cowboy threatens to let the Mantis dine on the dopey dean to make him work.

Ropes the dean early in the morning

Antipsychotics—The Crazy Library

"Did you hear something?!"
"Are you the President of the Universe?"
"Why **yes** I am!!!"

Whoa!!! Lost it for a second.

Introduction to Schizophrenia

Schizophrenia

    Characteristic disturbances:

        In perception ⇒ hallucinations and illusions

        In the form and content of thought ⇒ delusions

        In mood ⇒ usually flat or blunted affect, occasionally inappropriate

        In the sense of self and the relationship to the external world ⇒ loss of ego boundaries or social withdrawal

    Cause:

        The exact biochemical disturbances are yet to be delineated, but one theory is that it stems from excessive dopamine. The dopaminergic neurons that are responsible for this excess dopamine project from the ventral tegmental area of the mid brain to the limbic region of the neocortex.

    Treatment: Antipsychotic drugs, generally called neuroleptics, are thought to decrease psychotic symptoms by blocking the action of dopamine at the postsynaptic receptor (D2).

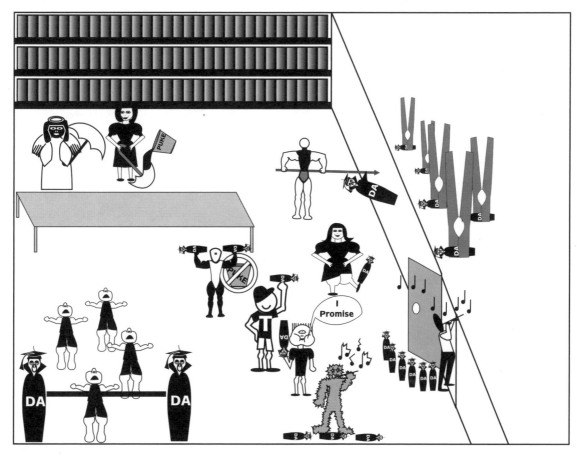

Picture Key

In this crazy picture, we remain at the Phunny Pharm University, but now the focus is upon a crazy party that is raging in the library. It is a "crazy" party because who ever thought of partying at the library anyway. At this party, psychotic people are doing the limbo while the limbo stick is held by the dopey dean. The antipsychotics (neuroleptics) cause the dopey dean to leave the party so it will calm down.

Dopamine—excess dopamine → psychosis
The <u>dopey dean vampire</u> holds the <u>limbo stick</u> and keeps the crazy party going in the library.

Psychosis
The <u>library</u> with the <u>crazy party</u> is normally a place for quiet study and thought, but is thrown into disorder by too much of the dopey dean.

Limbic areas of the brain
The <u>limbo</u> represents the limbic areas where the affected neurons project.

Dopamine receptors
The limbo stick is the receptor for the <u>dopey dean.</u>

Neuroleptics
Things that stop the dean from holding the stick or that make him leave the library.

Neuroleptics in General

N	Neuroleptics:	Things that take the dopey dean out of the library:
	Phenothiazines:	
	<u>Chlor</u>promazine	<u>Chlor</u> the cyclops <u>promising</u> to throw the dean out of the <u>scene</u>
	Trifluoperazine	A terrible musician <u>tries</u> to play the <u>flute</u>, and it causes the dean to <u>perish</u>.
	Fluphenazine	<u>Flute</u> player made the dean leave the <u>scene</u> with his music.
	Thioridazine	<u>Theo rids</u> the <u>scene</u> of the dean.
	Prochlorperazine	The <u>professional</u> cyclops named <u>Chlor</u> causes the dean to <u>perish</u>.
	Thiothixine	<u>Thighs</u> of a <u>thick</u> librarian kick the dean out.
	Atypicals:	
	Clozapine	<u>Clothespin</u> pins the dean down outside of the library, so he can't go in and stir things up.
	Risperidone	A w<u>rest</u>ler <u>spears</u> the <u>dean</u> and throws him out of the library.
	Butyrophenones:	
	Haloperidol	An angel who is wearing her <u>halo</u> and a <u>parasol</u>
	Droperidol	<u>Drops</u> her <u>parasol</u>
mech	??: block dopamine receptor in the meso<u>limbic</u> and mesocortical systems	The <u>dopey dean</u> is knocked off the <u>limbo stick</u> and out of the library by the neuroleptics.
Met	Liver metabolism—extensive first pass metabolism	They are put in jail.
$t_{1/2}$	Greater than 24 hrs	They can party for a long time.
Tox	Actually side effects, since the following occur at therapeutic doses: <u>D</u>epression <u>E</u>xtrapyramidal ⇒ movement disorders akathisia (restless legs), Parkinson's disease, and dystonic reaction <u>P</u>rolactinemia/<u>p</u>hotosensitivity <u>T</u>ardive dyskinesia <u>H</u>ypotension/<u>h</u>ypothalamic dysregulation Neuroleptic malignant syndrome	Their first letters spell <u>DEPTH</u> ⇒ They can get into deep trouble if they are too rough with the dean.
Rt	PO, IM, IV	

	IM for longer-lasting neuroleptics	
Uses	Schizophrenia and other psychosis	The crazy party at the library
	Antiemetics	They prevent hurling at the party when the dean leaves early.
	Delirium	

Phenothiazines

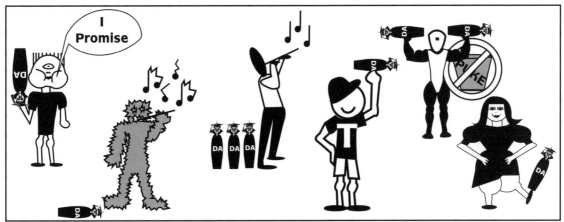

	Chlorpromazine **Trifluoperazine**	**Fluphenazine**	**Prochlorperazine** **Thioridazine** **Thiothixine**
N	All end in -zine		They are all ending the scene at the library when they throw the dean out:
	Chlorpromazine		Chlor the cyclops promising to throw the dean out of the scene
	Trifluoperazine		A terrible musician tries to play the flute, and it causes the dean to perish.
	Fluphenazine		Flute player made the dean leave the scene with his music.
	Thioridazine		Theo rids the scene of the dean.
	Prochlorperazine		The professional cyclops named Chlor causes the dean to perish.
	Thiothixine		Thighs of a thick librarian kick the dean out.
Tox	Sedation		The people in the library get tired after they throw the dean out.
	Reduction of seizure threshold		The dean gets mad when he has to leave the party ⇒ he shakes things up at the University.
Uses	Prochlorperazine ⇒ antiemetic		The professional cyclops named Chlor keeps the partiers in the library from throwing up.

Atypical Neuroleptics

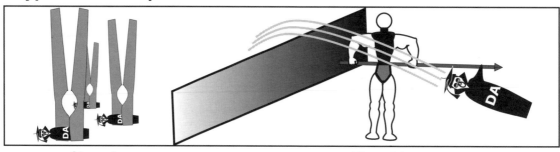

	Clozapine	**Risperidone**
N	<u>Clozapine</u>	A <u>clothespin</u> that pins the dean down outside of the library, so he can't go in and stir things up.
	<u>Risperidone</u>	A w<u>rest</u>ler <u>spears</u> the <u>dean</u> and throws him out of the library.
mech	Risperidone ⇒ blocks both dopamine and serotonin receptors	
Tox	Both have fewer extrapyramidal effects Clozapine ⇒ agranulocytosis	
Uses	Clozapine ⇒ may be useful when other antipsychotics have been ineffective	The clothespin is only used after the others have failed.

Butyrophenones

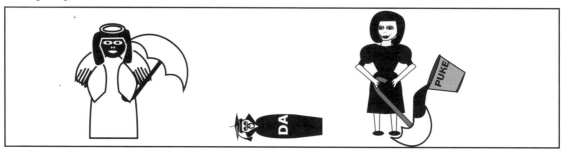

	Haloperidol	**Droperidol**
N	<u>Haloperidol</u>	An angel wearing her <u>halo</u> and a <u>parasol</u>
	<u>Droperidol</u>	<u>Drops</u> her <u>parasol</u> so she can use it to catch the vomit
Tox	Haldol ⇒ can have dramatic extrapyramidal effects	The angel can move you.
Uses	Haldol ⇒ Tourette's disease Huntington's disease Psychosis	
	<u>Droperidol</u> ⇒ antiemetic and anesthesia	She catches the vomit with her parasol.

Drugs That Alter Mood—The MAO Fraternity

Depression is the most prevalent psychiatric disorder and the cause of much suffering and loss of life. Exogenous depression, as the name implies, is provoked by an outside stimulus. It accounts for 60% of depression, and usually requires only short-term use of an antidepressant, if at all. In contrast, endogenous depression results from an internal imbalance. Generally, this is thought to be due to a deficiency of monoamine neurotransmitters (norepinephrine and/or serotonin) in the brain of the depressed patient.

Comparison Between Types of Major Depression

There are two types of major depression, unipolar and bipolar, and they are treated differently:

Unipolar depression:

Major depression—Patients plagued by fatigue, sadness, worthlessness, hopelessness, ↓ pleasure, loss of interest in usual activities, ↓ concentration, insomnia or hypersomnia, and thoughts of dying and suicide

Bipolar disease:

Cycle between major depression and manic or hypomanic episodes. These manic episodes are characterized by elevated mood, ↑ activity, pressured speech, grandiosity, distractibility, and involvement in dangerous activities, such as reckless driving and unsafe sex, which is normally uncharacteristic of these people.

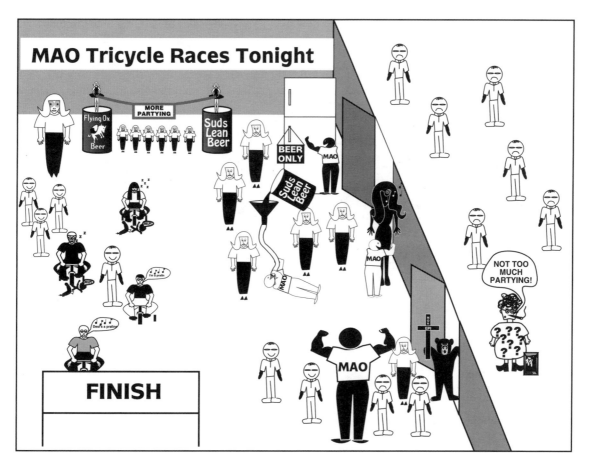

Dysthymia—Milder than major depression, but still can
    be incapacitating
Treatment: Tricyclic antidepressants, monoamine
    oxidase inhibitors (MAO) inhibitors, atypical
    antidepressants, and electroconvulsive therapy (ECT)

Treatment: lithium, valproate, carbamazepine,
    verapamil, clonazepam

Picture Key

    This picture takes us to the University of the Phunny Pharm, wherein we visit a party place. This place is the <u>M</u>u <u>A</u>lpha <u>O</u>mega Fraternity house. The antidepressants are people and things within the house that keep the party going. Please note that depression is a serious disease, and the association of a party with the treatment of the disease is not meant to belittle it.

Depression	People who are not partying
Bipolar disease	People who party too much → not at all → then too much again ⇒ those who are going in and out of the house
<u>M</u>onoamine <u>o</u>xidase <u>e</u>nzyme <u>s</u>ystem, which metabolizes norepinephrine and serotonin	The <u>bouncer</u> at the party who throws people out of the party when they have been there too long
<u>N</u>orepinephrine	Nick, the mean old bear, holding a cross with "<u>norepi</u>" written upon it. Nick uses the cross to make people happy.
<u>S</u>erotonin	<u>Sarah</u>, the party girl, who is <u>throw</u>ing the party and who keeps the party <u>going</u>

Antidepressants:
  Tricyclics
  Monoamine oxidase inhibitors
 	
  Atypical antidepressants
	Things that keep the party alive:
	  Tricycle races
	  Things that keep the bouncer from throwing people out of the party
	  The pledge class of the fraternity who are really into partying with Sarah only

Tricyclic Antidepressants (TCAs) in General

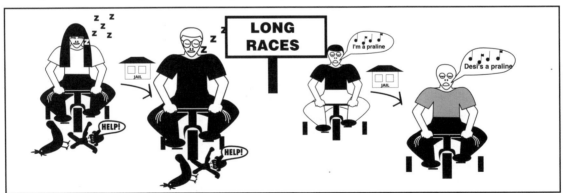

	Amitriptyline **Nortriptyline**	**Imipramine** **Desipramine**
N	Tricyclic antidepressants: <u>Amitriptyline</u> <u>Nortriptyline</u> <u>Imipramine</u> <u>Desipramine</u>	Tricycle races: <u>Am</u>y <u>rips to</u> the <u>line</u>. <u>Nor</u>ton <u>rips</u> to the <u>line</u>. He's singing "<u>I'm a praline</u>." <u>Desi</u> singing "<u>Desi's a praline</u>."
mech	Inhibit serotonin reuptake → ⇑ in serotonin levels in the CNS Inhibit norepinephrine reuptake → ⇑ in norepinephrine levels in the CNS	Races that convince Sarah to keep the party going Races that keep Nick the party bear with the norepi cross at the party to cheer people up.

Dist	90% protein bound	
Met	High first-pass liver metabolism	They can all go to jail.
	Amitriptyline is metabolized to nortryptyline	Amy gives Norton her tricycle.
	Imipramine is metabolized to desipramine	I'm gives his tricycle to Desi.
$t_{1/2}$	16–80 hr, but TCAs can take up to 2–3 wk to reach full effectiveness	Tricycles are very slow, and their races last a long time.
Tox	Anticholinergic side effects: dry mouth, tachycardia, constipation urinary retention, blurred vision. (Amitriptyline is the worst.)	The tricycle races distract the three musketeer cubs so they cannot get into mischief. They **cannot** slow down the train, poop, pee, or see.
	Cardiac:	
	Postural hypotension	
	Arrhythmias—V tach and fibrillation	
	CNS:	The University:
	Fever, seizures, coma	Tricycle racers can get hot, shaky, and comatose.
	If "ipramine" is in the name of the tricyclic, it is less sedating than other tricyclics.	These are too busy saying "I'm a praline" and "Desi's a praline" to run over the rooster.
	May → manic episode.	Tricyclists can make depressed people party too much.
	TCAs take up to 2–3 wk to reach full effectiveness ⇒ patients may discontinue due to lack of improvement	Tricycles are very slow.
	Dangerous in overdoses	
Rt	All PO	
Uses	Major depressive (unipolar) disorder	Only unhappy people can be cheered up by tricycle races.
	Pain control: peripheral neuropathies, trigeminal neuralgia, and cancer; also treats the depression associated with these diseases	A tricycle can be used to disconnect the rest of the Phunny Pharm from the University weather station.*
	Sedation	The tricycle racer runs over the rooster responsible for keeping the Phunny Pharm awake.†

Monoamine Oxidase Inhibitors

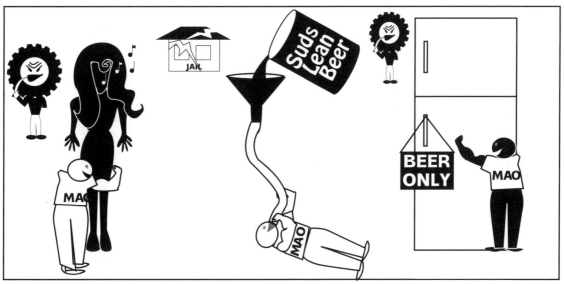

Tranylcypromine	Phenelzine	Isocarboxazid

---

*Rem: The University weather station represents the sensation of pain throughout the Phunny Pharm.
†Rem: Please see chapter on sedatives/hypnotics, where the reticular activating system (RAS) is a rooster keeping the farmer awake.

N	Monoamine oxidase inhibitors:	Things that distract the bouncer:
	Tranylcypromine	Entrancing siren
	Phenelzine	Funnel for a beer bong
	Isocarboxazid	Ice box with beer in it
mech	Inhibit monoamine oxidase, which metabolizes monoamines such as dopamine, norepinephrine, and serotonin → ↑d levels of dopamine, norepinephrine, and serotonin → elevated mood	All these things keep the bouncer from doing his job, such that he can't throw Sarah the party gal and the norepi cross out of the party → they allow Sarah and the norepi cross to keep the party going.
	Also inhibits oxidases usually responsible for metabolism of drugs and tyramine-containing foods → ↑ tyramine (a sympathomimetic) ⇒ see Tox	There is another bouncer at the beach* who is responsible for guarding the entrance to the Phunny Pharm. He is also distracted by these → too much of the tire man in the Phunny Pharm.
Tox	Hypertensive crisis with cheddar cheese, beer, wine, amphetamines, alphamethyl dopa, L-dopa, and decongestants	With the bouncer distracted, the tire man has free run of the body.
	Hepatic necrosis	These things break the jail.
Rt	PO	
Uses	Major depression	¢: These are for depression.
	Dysthymia	
	Failure of TCAs	If the tricycle races aren't any fun, it still can be fun to watch the bouncer get messed up.
	Narcolepsy	
	Parkinson's disease	¢: Also ↑ dopamine levels.
	Phobic/anxiety states	It's relaxing to watch the bouncer distracted.

Atypical or Second-Generation Antidepressants

The second-generation antidepressants are a diverse group of medicines often called atypical antidepressants. Their mechanisms vary if they're known at all, but they are thought to increase amine levels in the CNS. The ones that are in the Phunny Pharm are selective serotonin reuptake inhibitors (SSRIs). They can be used as first-line antidepressants for major depression.

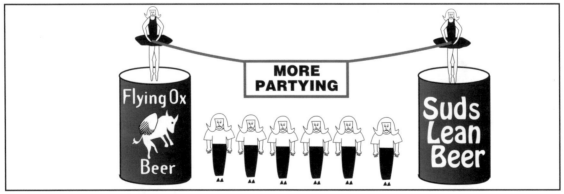

	Fluoxetine	**Sertraline**
N	Selective serotonin reuptake inhibitors:	Only Sarah drinks beer:
	Fluoxetine	Flying Ox beer
	Sertraline	Suds Lean beer
mech	Selectively block serotonin reuptake	Flying Ox beer and Suds Lean beer are Sarah's favorites. They keep her at the party.
$t_{1/2}$	2–3 d	She stays for days for the beer.

*Rem: The beach is the "entrance to the Phunny Pharm" (i.e., the sight where the oral medicines enter the body).

Tox	No anticholinergic properties, little cardiovascular effect	The three musketeer cubs are not stopped by the beer.
	Nausea, headache, nervousness, insomnia, diarrhea	You can get a hangover with these beers, however.
Uses	Major depression	The beer keeps Sarah the party girl partying.
	Obsessive/compulsive disorder	She is less obsessive when she is drinking beer.

Another Serotonin Reuptake Inhibitor

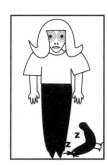

	Trazodone	**Trance Is Done on Sarah**
mech	Primary effect is mediated by inhibition of serotonin reuptake	Sarah is in a trance ⇒ she can't leave the party.
Tox	Most sedating antidepressant	The trance puts the rooster to sleep.
	Priapism (persistent erection)	Forget it!! You come up with something.
	No anticholinergic effects	Three musketeer cubs are not affected by the trance.
Rt	PO	
Uses	Aggressive disorders	

Bipolar Disease

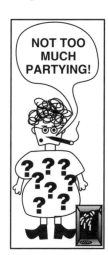

	Lithium	**Letha "The House Mother"**
mech	?????	
	Lithium prevents mood swings and slows cycling between depression and mania.	Letha keeps the party at the frat house from becoming too wild (manic), but still lets everyone have fun.
Met	Kidney	She goes to the showers when she is through.
Tox	Initial:	When the house mother is first hired, her cooking sucks, so everyone's stomach hurts, they are thirsty, they get tired of her food, and their hands shake as they force the food to their mouths.
	GI disturbance	
	Thirst	
	Fatigue	
	Sedation	
	Hand tremors	
	Later:	After a while, her cooking gets better, but the food lacks salt (everyone got goiters).
	Goiter	
	Diabetes insipidus	
	Lithium toxicity is ↑ with low sodium chloride ingestion.	Her cooking is much worse when there is a shortage of salt.
Rt	PO (as a salt)	She is a cook.
R_x/R_x	Caffeine ⇒ ↓ lithium levels	Letha would rather drink coffee than stay at the party ⇒ she leaves the party when there is coffee available.
	NSAIDs ⇒ ↑ lithium levels	Letha hates sailing ⇒ when there are sailboats around she stays at the party.*

---

*Rem: The NSAIDs are sailboats.

Narcotic Analgesics—The University's Big-O Bar

The narcotic analgesics or opiates are a group of naturally occurring, semisynthetic, and synthetic compounds that have been used for centuries to reduce pain. They exert their effects by interacting with several types of opiate receptors. The functions of these receptors have not been completely delineated for their pharmacologic importance.

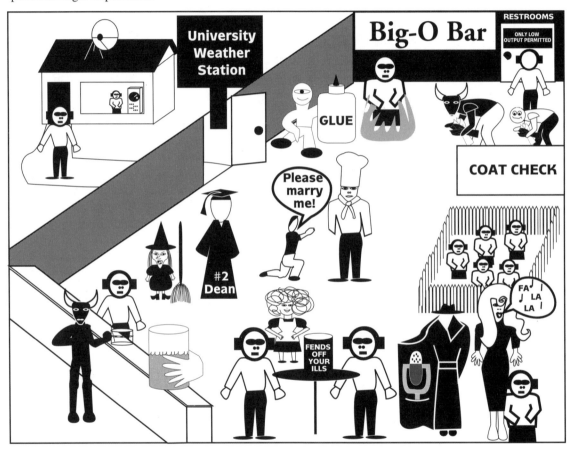

Picture Key

In this picture, we remain in the University, but we return briefly to the weather station to look into the weather around the Phunny Pharm. If there is a bad storm with damage, the weather station monitors it. If the damage is severe, then we can help the weather people by taking them to the Big-O Bar and distracting them from the pain of destruction.

Pain	Weather damage to the Phunny Pharm that is "sensed" by the weather station
Normal response to pain	The weather station can mobilize the University to do something about the destruction.
Severe pain	Severe destruction in the Phunny Pharm due to a bad storm. When the weather people see this much damage, it is very painful to them.

| Pain relief | Prevent the weather people from seeing the damage. |
| Narcotic analgesics | Things that prevent the weather people from seeing the damage by taking them to the Big-O Bar |

Full Agonists

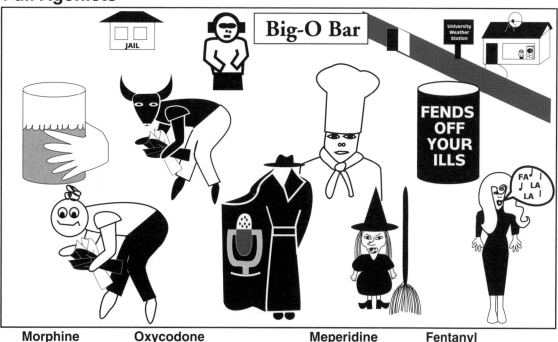

Morphine   Oxycodone
Hydrocodone   Hydromorphone   Methadone
Meperidine   Fentanyl
Sufentanil

N	Morphine	If they are given <u>more fingers</u>, they will remain at the bar longer*.
	Hydrocodone	<u>Hider</u> of <u>coats</u> hides the weather peoples' coats so they cannot go back to the weather station.
	Oxycodone	An <u>ox</u> who takes <u>coats</u> and prevents the people from leaving
	Hydromorphone	A person who <u>hides</u> a <u>microphone</u>, sings, and has a good time → they stay longer
	Meperidine	"<u>Me</u> perfect <u>dinner</u>" is a chef who cooks for the weather people and helps to keep them at the bar.
	Methadone	<u>Martha dons</u> her broom and sweeps the narcotic addicts into the bar where shelter can be found.
	Fentanyl	A drink that <u>fends</u> off your <u>ills</u>
	Sufentanil	Sue <u>fends</u> off your <u>ills</u>; she is the bar singer.
mech	Agonists at opiate receptors → elevate pain threshold and change response to pain	They are at the bar and distract the weather people from the pain of the weather damage.
Met	Liver metabolism	If they get too rowdy at the Big-O Bar, they will go to jail.
	Glucuronidation and urinary excretion	
$t_{1/2}$	Methadone ⇒ longer onset and duration of action than others	

---

*A "finger" is a measurement used to denote that the amount of alcohol in the drink is a finger width.

Tox	Behavioral effects: euphoria, hallucinations, sedation, lethargy, confusion	People in bars act strange.
	Depression of respiration	Because the weather people are not at their station, they cannot monitor the weather for the airport, and the movement of air traffic slows down.
	Nausea and vomiting	¢: They directly → release of histamine in the GI tract → stimulation and nausea
	Miosis except for meperidine	The three musketeer cubs are by the closed eye caves.
	Constipation	Plugs 'em up so they remain in the bathroom of the bar
	Urinary retention	Plugs 'em up so they can't pee
	Tolerance	The weather people get tired of the bar, and it takes more to keep them distracted.
	Dependence	
	Meperidine → seizures	The chief causes are earthquakes
Uses	Analgesia	¢: From mechanism of action
	Pain of malignancy	
	Painful diagnostic procedures	
	Postoperative medication	
	Obstetric anesthesia	
	Post MI	
	Cough suppression	Helps them endure tickling in their throats better
	Antidiarrheals	¢: Constipation is a side effect.
	End-stage pulmonary edema	
	Methadone ⇒ treatment of narcotic addiction because it is taken PO and has less euphoria	Martha sweeps the narcotic addicts off of the street and into the bar.
	Fentanyl ⇒ anesthesia	

Full Agonist Used Chiefly for Antidiarrheal Effects

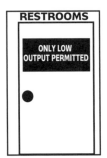

	Loperamide		**Only <u>Low</u> Output <u>Permitted</u>**
N	<u>Loperamide</u>		A sign on the bathroom door reading, << Only <u>Low</u> Output <u>Permitted</u> >>
Dist	Very poorly absorbed from GI tract		¢: As this is only used for diarrhea.
Uses	Antidiarrheal		¢

Partial or Weak Agonists

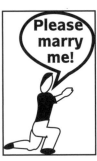

	Propoxyphene		**The <u>Proposal Fiend</u>**
N	<u>Propoxyphene</u>		The <u>proposal fiend</u> runs around the bar proposing to marry everyone.
mech	Weak agonist, less potent than aspirin		This is weakly humorous to watch, so the weather people will remain at the bar.
Tox	Dizziness, sedation, nausea, and vomiting		¢: These are basically the same as for the full agonist.
	In overdose ⇒ CNS depression, convulsions, coma, death		
Rt	PO		
Uses	Minor pain relief		Only helps with minimal weather damage

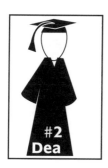

Codeine

N   Codeine

mech   A prodrug; 10% is converted to morphine

Uses   Minor pain relief

        Antitussive

The Co-Dean of the University

The co-dean of the University goes to the Big-O Bar when there is weather damage to help calm people down.

He helps to keep people at the bar by giving them a couple of fingers in their drinks. He does not give them as many fingers as more fingers.

The few fingers that he gives the people are enough for minor damage and to prevent the tickling in their throats.

Antagonists

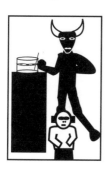

Naloxone

N   Naloxone

Dist   Not available orally

Uses   Treatment of opiate overdose

        Reversal of acute effects of opiates

        Reversal of effects of endogenous opiates

The New Ox Bartender

The new ox bartender's only job is to keep you safe. If you have had a few too many, he will kick you out.

Doesn't talk much

If the weather people begin to get the effects of too much time at the bar, he will kick them out.

He kicks all of the weather people out of the bar.

He will even kick the normal residents of the bar out.

Mixed Agonist–Antagonists

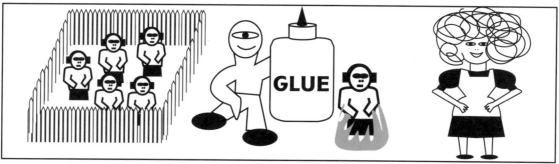

Pentazocine	**Nalbuphine**	**Butorphanol**

N   Pentazocine   Pens the weather people at the scene.

      Nalbuphine   A new glue fiend who glues the weather people to the floor of the bar

      Butorphanol   The beautiful orphan waitress

mech   Have both agonistic and antagonistic actions at opiate receptors   These are the service people for the Big-O Bar, such that they "go-between" the bartender and the customers (i.e., their job is to distract the customer, but at the same time they cannot go overboard).

Tox	Less respiratory depression	They all used to be flight attendants, so they have a special place in their hearts for the airplanes and wouldn't jeopardize their safety.
	May increase cardiac work	They may make your heart pound.
	Dysphoria:	
	Pentazocine $\Rightarrow$ higher incidence of dysphoric effects	
	Nalbuphine $\Rightarrow$ less dysphoria than pentazocine	
Uses	Analgesia when less than maximum efficacy and greater safety is required	They will let you party, but part of their job is to keep you safe: "Our primary responsibility is your safety. Thank you for flying with Big-O."

General Anesthesia—The Airport and Planes That Bomb the University

These medications are very important in today's practice of medicine—important enough that a specialty exists that is devoted entirely to their administration and the safety of the anesthetized patient.

Anesthetic Definitions

Anesthesia	Lack of ALL feeling
General	The loss of consciousness
Regional	Loss of all feeling in a region of the body
Analgesia	Relief from pain
Muscle relaxation	

Mechanism of Action

Although many theories have been proposed, the mechanism of anesthetics is not yet certain. It is apparent that the action of the anesthetic is correlated with the partial pressure in the brain (PP_{brain}), and the membranes of the cells are the most likely site of action.

Characteristics of Anesthetics

Uncharged, nonpolar, and unrelated to each other

They do not act by direct interaction with a receptor $\Rightarrow$ no antagonists to their actions

Nonspecific in their actions

Site of Action

Hydrophobic portions of the cells, including membranes and certain sites in proteins

Actions in the hydrophobic area cause a change in lipid: protein interactions and thereby alter ion currents across membranes

In the brain, inhibitory ionic currents are enhanced and excitatory currents are inhibited. In this, at least one site of action seems to be the GABA channels

Distribution

The main trick in dealing with general anesthetics is getting the drug to the brain. Although this is a subject that may be left for an anesthesia rotation and for some reason is not covered in the study guides that I have seen, it is a concept that is easy to understand using the pictures that have been used throughout the Phunny Pharm. If the distribution of anesthetics during induction and maintenance of anesthesia is not covered in your course, then skip this section; however, you may find it useful to return to this section before your anesthesia rotation.

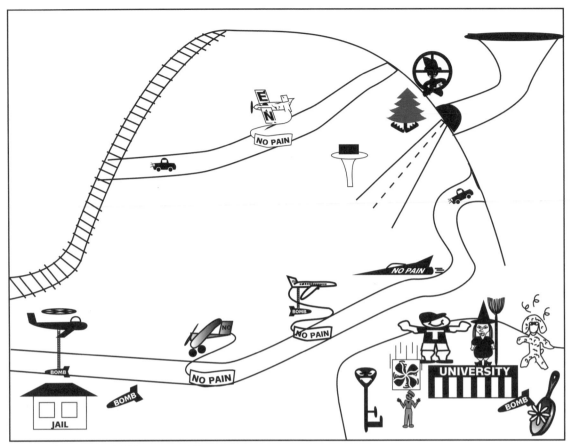

Physics and Picture Key

Most general anesthetics are gases and therefore are most easily administered through the lungs. In the following discussion, **"gas" will be used only to refer to the physical state (gas), whereas "anesthetic" will be used to refer to the drug or anesthetic.** This is essential to keep straight!

Inhaled anesthetics	Planes
Lungs	A series of tubes through which planes fly on their way to the airports
Alveoli	Airports
The vasculature in the body	Roads
Brain	The CNS University*
Anesthesia	A plane's ability to destroy the University, measured by the type of bomb or the weight that it can carry
Analgesia	The planes carry a sign that explain their analgesic ability.
Muscle relaxation	The year of medical school in which the pilot is enrolled: 1st yr ⇒ no relaxation; 2nd yr ⇒ some relaxation; 4th yr ⇒ very good relaxation

In any fluid, there are **two** forms of an anesthetic:
1. The portion in <u>solution</u> (i.e., dissolved in the blood)
2. The portion that remains as a <u>gas</u>, which is measured by partial pressure (PP)

Planes can fly or drive:
1. The planes that <u>drive</u> on the road are in solution.
2. The planes and other things that <u>fly</u> above the roads are in the gaseous state.

---

*Rem: The CNS is represented by the University throughout the Phunny Pharm.

Solubility of anesthetic in the blood:

Preference of planes to drive or fly:
High solubility ⇒ few planes in the air, many on the roads
Low solubility ⇒ many planes in the air, few on the roads

Partial pressure (PP):
This is the only portion of the drug that contributes to anesthesia and analgesia.

Number of planes that are flying in that area

Blood/gas solubility (lambda = λ):
The more soluble the gas, the more gas that enters solution, and therefore does not contribute to the PP.

Preference of planes to drive on the road instead of fly. The more that prefer to drive, instead of fly, leaves fewer in the air.*

Minimum alveolar concentration (MAC):
A measurement of potency for general anesthetics ⇒ 1MAC = inhaled concentration at which 50% of people do not respond to a surgical incision.

The number of planes that need to be flown into the body to get the job done. If fewer planes are needed, then it is a more "potent plane."

Steps of Distribution

In order to achieve anesthesia, the drug is inhaled into the lung at a set concentration (i.e., PP). This equilibrates across the alveoli with the blood. The rate at which this occurs depends upon its solubility. If the drug is very soluble in blood, then the PPs will not equilibrate, as the PP_{blood} will always be less than the PP_{lung}. The drug is then carried via the blood to the brain, in which it equilibrates again and obtains its own partial pressure. Then an equilibrium occurs, such that the "steady state" ($PP_{lung} = PP_{blood} = PP_{brain}$) exists. It must be noticed that because concentration = PP + Drug in Solution, at steady state only the PPs are equal, whereas the concentrations are not.

"Lung washout": The concentration of gas in the lungs (C_A) approaches the inspired concentration (C_I). With each breath of gas at C_I, the anesthetic entering the lung is diluted by the gas already in the lung. With more breaths, the concentration of anesthetic in the lungs increases toward C_I.

The planes fly through tubes to get to the airports. At the airports, they have more room to fly initially, since there are few planes in a large area. With each additional wave of planes, there are more left from the previous wave. Eventually, the airport will have the same maneuvering space as in the tubes.

Anesthetic uptake by pulmonary blood: (A constant "leak" that prevents $C_I = C_A$) Uptake into the blood is determined by the blood flow and the solubility of the anesthetic in the blood.

The maneuvering of the planes onto the roads of the body. This is determined by the speed at which they can fly with the road, and the number of them that are not flying above the road.

Uptake of anesthetic by the body:
Rate of uptake by the body is determined by the blood flow to the tissue and the tissue's solubility for the anesthetic. High blood flow has the highest initial uptake ⇒ the brain.
Rate is also determined by the PP of anesthetic that remains when the blood arrives at the tissue.

The number of planes that can fly into the tissue is determined by how big the roads are that go to the tissue and how welcome the planes are in that tissue.
Rate is also determined by the number of planes that are still flying above the ground when they get to the tissue.

Tissue redistribution:
This is the main factor in emergence from general anesthesia after administration is stopped.

---

*Note: λ sounds like "lander," so that the higher λ is, the more the planes want to land on the roads and drive.

General Anesthetics in General

Because the ability of each anesthetic to produce anesthesia, analgesia, and muscle relaxation is one of the main points to remember in this chapter, please notice that I have added three new sections to the tables.

mech	The perfect anesthetic (none have all five):	The perfect plane would have:
	1. → Unconsciousness	1. A large payload to temporarily destroy the University
	2. → Analgesia	2. A sign that says "No Pain," and prevents things from falling upon the University
	3. → Muscle relaxation	3. A fourth-year medical student pilot
	4. → Rapid induction and emergence from anesthesia	4. Would not want to drive on the road; would only want to fly
	5. Wide therapeutic index	5. No damage to the University
Met	Since these drugs are relatively inert, they are not extensively metabolized.	
Tox	Drugs that are metabolized by the liver → toxicities secondary to production of the metabolites.	If the plane is a police plane, then it may cause more toxicities.
	Respiratory depression such that patients are usually intubated and respirations are controlled	
	Cardiovascular depression	
Rt	Inhalation	Represented by things that can fly

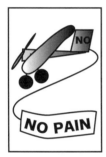

		Nitrous Oxide	**Ultra Light with NO on the Tail**
	Anesth	Low potency ⇒ only get complete anesthesia at hyperbaric pressures.	Can carry only a small payload ⇒ small bombs
	Analg	Excellent	It is pulling a large sign that says "No Pain."
	Relax	None	A second-year medical student just before boards is flying this plane.
	mech	Very insoluble in blood (low λ)	This plane does not want to land and drive, because it will get run over by other cars.
	Tox	"Second gas effect" ⇒ hypoxia during arousal from anesthesia. Because of the insolubility of nitrous oxide (NO) in blood, it is rapidly excreted back into lungs → hypoxia as it displaces O_2 in the alveoli.	The pilot must wear O_2 mask to prevent possible hypoxia.
	Uses	Adjunct with other agents for its analgesic activity	Since the ultra light has a small payload, it needs help in an attack on the University
		Also for minor procedures with a regional analgesic	

Halogenated Hydrocarbons in General

N	Halothane, isoflurane, enflurane, and methoxyflurane	Helo-plane, ISO Airlines, EN plane, and the foxy fighter plane.
mech	Halogens → decreased flammability and toxicity seen in "historical" anesthetics (diethyl ether and chloroform)	
Uses	Usually used with muscle relaxants secondary to minimal relaxation	Only the ISO Airlines and the EN plane are flown by a fourth-year medical student.

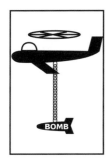

Halothane

Anesth	Good
Analg	Poor
Relax	Fair
Met	Metabolized by the liver to an extent
Tox	Malignant hyperthermia:
	"Halothane hepatitis" secondary to sensitivity to metabolites
Uses	Good anesthesia, but lacks analgesia and muscle relaxation

Helicopter Plane (Helo-Plane)

A big helicopter that can lift large payloads, and it is carrying a large bomb

The sign it is pulling is burning.

A first-year medical student is flying the helo-plane.

The helo-plane is a police helicopter, so it will follow orders from the police station to land.*

The helo-plane may overheat and crash.

The helo-plane may crash into the police department when it lands there.

¢

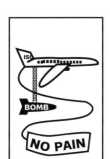

Isoflurane

Anesth	Good
Analg	Good
Relax	Good
Tox	No hepatic or renal toxicity

ISO Airline Plane

Can carry a large payload

It is pulling a sign that says "No Pain."

Piloted by a fourth year medical student

No damage to the jail or shower

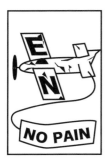

Enflurane

Anesth	Fair
Analg	Good
Relax	Good
Tox	Seizures

EN Old Plane

Can carry small loads ⇒ it is old.

It is pulling a "No Pain" sign.

Piloted by a fourth-year medical student

This plane is so old that it shakes.

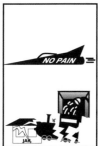

Methoxyflurane

Anesth	Very good
Analg	Very good
Tox	Profound respiratory and circulatory depression
	Fluoride toxicity → renal failure
	Does not relax uterus
Uses	Only used in special circumstances, including obstetrics, secondary to toxicities

Foxy Fighter Plane

Carries a large payload and can use nuclear bombs

Has sign on its fuselage saying "No Pain"

It flies so fast that it may miss the University and blow up the train, the airport, or the shower at the end of the trail.†

<<Top secret—special operations only>>

---

*Rem: The liver is represented by the Police department throughout The Phunny Pharm.
†Rem: The kidney is represented by the shower at the end of the trail throughout The Phunny Pharm.

General Anesthesia Adjuncts

Ultra-Short–Acting Barbiturates

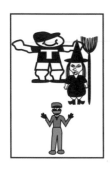

Thiopental and Methohexital

Anesth	Very good
Dist	Very large secondary to high <u>lipid</u> solubility
$t_{1/2}$	Rapid onset of action; also rapid emergence from anesthesia secondary to rapid redistribution to less vascularized tissues having high fat content
Tox	Cardiovascular and respiratory depression
Uses	<u>Induction</u> of anesthesia by IV

Theo Pens Them All and Martha Hexes Them All

Relaxes them all so much that they lose consciousness

¢ They are both <u>fat</u>

¢

¢: From the rapid onset of action

Other IV Anesthetics

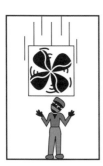

Propofol

mech	Anesthesia by unknown mechanism
Tox	Decreases systemic arterial pressure
Uses	Induction and maintenance of anesthesia

Falling Propeller

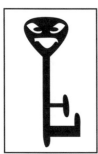

Ketamine

Analg	Good
Tox	Hallucinations and nightmares upon recovery
	No respiratory depression but can increase blood pressure and cardiac output
Uses	"Dissociative anesthetic" Superficial pain only Amnesia Primarily used in children

The Key to Mean Operations

It is the key to mean operations. Although it is the key to mean operations, it is also the key to mean dreams.

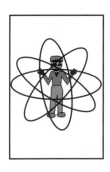

Etomidate

mech   Hypnotic without analgesia

Tox   Does not usually cause
respiratory or cardiovascular
depression

            Involuntary muscle movements

<u>Atom</u> for Surgery

Benzodiazepines

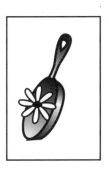

Diazepam

$t_{1/2}$ Long onset of action

Uses   Anxiolytic prior to surgery

       Anterograde amnesia and sedation

<u>Daisies in a Pan</u>

Patients getting ready for an operation
may get daisies to help them relax.

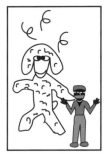

Midazolam

$t_{1/2}$ Faster onset and recovery than with
diazepam

Uses   Amnesia

<u>My Daisy</u> Eating a <u>Lamb</u>

This daisy eats the lamb faster than
daisies in the pan.

Analgesics

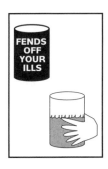

<u>Fenta</u>nyl and <u>Morphine</u>

mech   Narcotic analgesic

Tox   Respiratory depression

A Drink That <u>Fends</u> off Your <u>Ills</u> and the Drink with <u>More Fingers</u>

They are both found in the Big-O Bar.

They make the weather people of the
weather station not worry about the
weather at the airport.

Anticholinergics

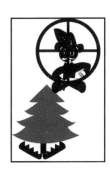

<u>Atropine</u> and <u>Scopolamine</u>

mech   Anticholinergic → blockade of
parasympathetic tone on the heart,
and reduce secretions

<u>A Trap in the Pine</u> and <u>a Scope</u> Fixed on the Cubs

They both prevent the three
musketeer cubs from slowing the
heart and from making secretions.

Muscle Paralysis

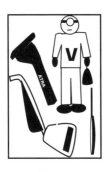

Pancuronium, Vecuronium, Atracurium, and Succinylcholine

mech   Block neuromuscular junction → muscular relaxation.

Rt   IV

The Pan, Vet, Atra Razor, and Vaccuum That Sucks

The pan, vet, Atra razor, and vaccuum that sucks prevent Nicky the bear from working out at the NM Junction Gym.

Antiemetics

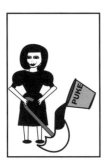

Droperidol

mech   Antiemetic by dopamine antagonism

Drops Her Parasol

She catches the vomit with her parasol.

Local Anesthetics—Shorting the Wires Monitoring Weather

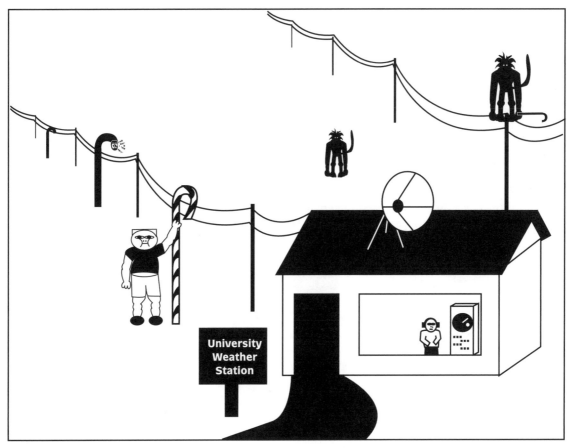

Picture Key

Pain that is sensed in the CNS is pictured as a weather station that monitors the weather (pain) throughout the Phunny Pharm. When pain is seen in the body, it mobilizes the University to respond to the pain.

CNS	The Phunny Pharm University
Pain	Bad weather in the Phunny Pharm ⇒ damage is occurring
Sensory nerves that transport pain signals from the periphery to the brain	The wires that carry the signal from the storm-damaged area to the weather station
Local anesthetics	Canes that sever the connection between the weather station and the Phunny Pharm
Uncharged base form of the anesthetic	When the canes are in the pocket of the climber, they are uncharged.
Charged acid form of the anesthetic	After the climber climbs the pole, he takes the cane out of his pocket (it is charged) and uses it to short out the wires.
Movement of drug into the nerve cells as an uncharged base	Movement of cane up the pole while in the pocket of the climber

Local Anesthetics in General

	Lidocaine	Procaine	Bupivacaine
N	Lidocaine		A little cain used to short out the wires running to the University.
	Procaine		A profane cane that shorts out the wires.
	Bupivacaine		The little pupil's cane that is used to short the wires running to the University.
mech	**Interfere with neuronal conduction of pain signals to the brain:**		The canes short the wires running to the University, so that the weather station cannot see the storm.
	Procaine is an ester. Lidocaine and bupivacaine are amides.		
	They exist as the uncharged base and the charged acid.*		They all can either be in the climber's pocket (uncharged) or out of the pocket (charged).
	The uncharged base form of the anesthetic moves across the neuronal cell membrane.		When they are in the climber's pocket, they can move up or down the pole.
	In the basic environment of the axonal cytoplasm, the base loses its H^+ and becomes charged.		At the top of the pole, the climber takes the cane out and uses it to short out the wire.
	The charged acid **binds the Na^+ channel** $\rightarrow$ blockade of the channel $\rightarrow$ failure of Na channel to respond to an action potential $\rightarrow$ loss of neuronal conduction.		They use the cane to short out the wire.
Dist	Concomitant administration of a vasoconstrictor agent, $\downarrow$ systemic absorption.		Things that close down the roads, prevent the canes and profanity from leaking to the rest of the Phunny Pharm
Met	Esters are metabolized by pseudocholinesterase and urine secretion. Amides are metabolized by liver.		
$t_{1/2}$	Lidocaine < procaine < bupivacaine		The canes are these lengths in order.
Tox	Only occur with higher doses and dependent upon systemic absorption: CNS $\Rightarrow$ can cause CNS depression and convulsions.		¢: Larger doses are required before they leak out into the rest of the body. If the canes get into the University, they will short out lots of things, making people depressed and causing explosions at the University.
	CV $\Rightarrow$ generalized vasodilation, $\downarrow$ in inotropy $\rightarrow$ $\downarrow$ cardiac output and hypotension.		Canes can cause $\downarrow$ blood pressure.

*Rem: The acid and base are pairs in that they can be converted from one to the other by the equation $LA + H^+ \leftrightarrow HLA^+$, where LA is the uncharged base form of the local anesthetic and HLA^+ is the charged acid form of the local anesthetic.

Cardiovascular System—The Train and Roads of the Phunny Pharm

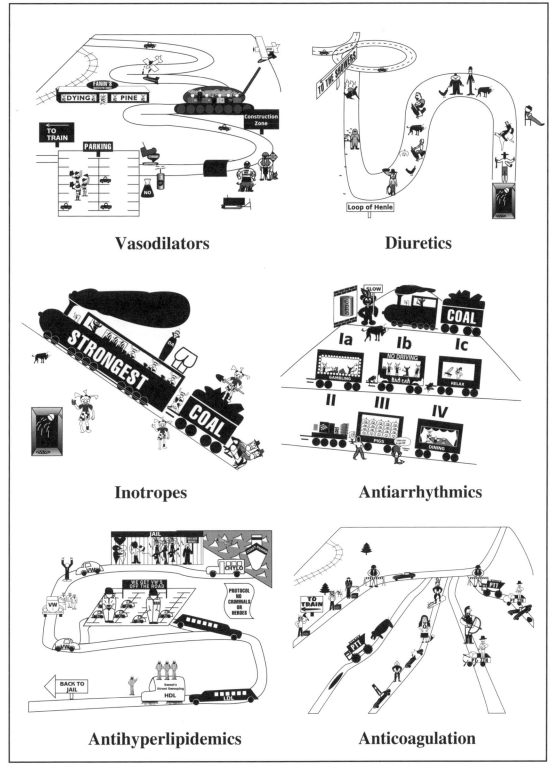

Vasodilators

Diuretics

Inotropes

Antiarrhythmics

Antihyperlipidemics

Anticoagulation

Picture Key

This picture takes us to the roads that appear in many pictures of the Phunny Pharm. It represents a series of roads that connect the different parts of the body.

Blood vessels	Roads
Blood	Cars and anything that can be found on roads
Myocardium	Engines that pull the train up the hill
Sarcomere of the myocardial cell	Each individual engine
<u>Afterload</u>: Pressure gradient that must be overcome to pump the blood out of the heart	"Afterload Hill," which the train must climb
Rhythm	The engineers of the train
Diastole	The time at the bottom of the hill when the cars and animals get onto the train
Systole	The time it takes the train to move up "Afterload Hill" and let the cars and animals off the train at the top
At the top of the pressure gradient, the pressure begins to decrease	After the top of "Afterload Hill," the cars get off the train and coast down the hill on the roads
<u>K</u>idney	The <u>sh</u>ower at the end of the Phunny Pharm cattle drive trail
<u>W</u>ater	<u>Fl</u>ies: They follow the animals wherever they go.
<u>S</u>odium	<u>S</u>teers*
<u>P</u>otassium	<u>P</u>igs
Proton (i.e., <u>h</u>ydrogen ions)	<u>H</u>ogs
<u>Ch</u>loride	<u>Ch</u>ickens
<u>B</u>icarbonate, which can undergo dehydration to <u>C</u>O$_2$ (the gaseous state)	<u>B</u>ees in the hive ⇒ bicarbonate is represented by an animal that CAN <u>fl</u>y because it can be converted to a gaseous state. When they are in solution (i.e., bicarbonate), the bees are in the hive.
<u>C</u>alcium	<u>C</u>ows†: Milk is high in calcium.

Physiology

Although it is not my goal to review the cardiovascular physiology in detail, the following is a brief review of the system in a framework that will aid in the recollection of the important properties of the drugs.

Purpose Analogy

Cardiovascular system	Delivery of O$_2$ and other things to the periphery	The series of roads and the train
Heart	Pumps blood	The train that hauls things up "Afterload Hill"
Blood vessels	Keep blood organized	The roads and places for cars to drive
Arterioles	Maintain blood pressure by creating resistance at periphery	The roads: There are usually a shortage of lanes that cause a lot of traffic in these areas.
Veins	Blood reservoir	The parking lots

Cardiac Output

Anyone who has exercised realizes that the heart changes its functional capacity to accommodate the changing needs of the body. The heart does this by controlling the amount of blood it pumps, the cardiac output (CO):

$$CO \text{ (cardiac output)} = SV \text{ (stroke volume)} \times HR \text{ (heart rate)}$$

This equation makes sense because increasing either of these variables will increase the amount of blood pumped by the heart. Changes in both can be felt with exercise ⇒ your heart beats harder (an increase in SV) and you become tachycardic (an increase in HR); therefore, CO increases.

---

*Rem: A steer is a castrated male bovine.

†Rem: A cow is a female bovine.

Stroke Volume

First, stroke volume is exactly what the name implies, the volume of blood pumped with each stroke of the heart, or

$$\text{Stroke volume} = \text{volume at end of diastole} - \text{volume at end of systole}$$

Therefore, the determinants of SV are the "fullness" of the ventricle prior to contraction (governed by volume of blood returning to the heart) and the fraction of that volume the heart is able to eject (governed by preload, afterload, and contractility of the heart).

Preload

Preload can be defined by many things. It is the ventricular pressure just prior to contraction (i.e., precontraction). Because the pressure in the ventricle at rest is proportional to the volume, preload can also be represented by the end-diastolic volume. Because the volume in the heart stretches the ventricular walls, preload is also the stretch placed upon the sarcomeres. In the simplest terms, **preload** is the mechanism by which the heart changes its function to ensure that the volume **into** the heart always **equals** the volume **leaving** the heart. This is an intrinsic property, as it is one that is built into the design of the heart.

Afterload

Afterload, in the simplest terms, is the pressure against which the blood must be pumped, or the ease with which the blood moves. This property also determines the tension that develops in the wall of the heart prior to ejection of the blood.

Contractility

Contractility is the strength of the myocardium.

Vasodilators—Enlarge Roads

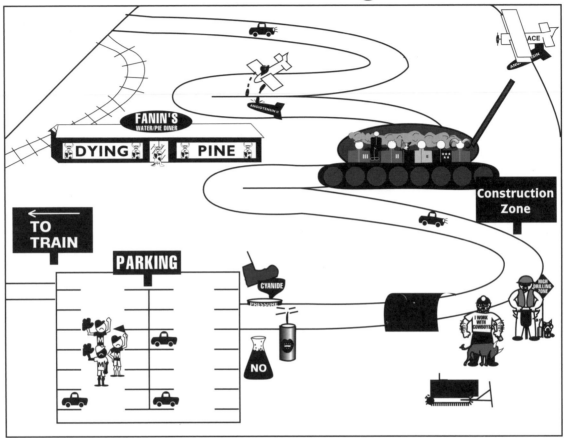

Picture Key: The Phunny Pharm Highway

In this picture, we remain on the roads of the Phunny Pharm. Anything that is seen destroying roads causes hypertension, and anything that makes roads or prevents the destruction of these roads decreases blood pressure.

Arteries	Roads leading to smaller roads
Arterioles	Smaller roads leading to parking lots
Veins	Parking lots
Calcium	Mean cows that run around and close roads
Heart	The Phunny Pharm train
Angiotensin converting enzyme	The ACE fighter pilot
Angiotensin II	The <<angiotensin II>> bomb being dropped by the ACE fighter pilot

Direct-Acting Vasodilators in General

N	Hydralazine, trimethaphan, nitrates, minoxidil, diazoxide	HTN M.D. ⇒ Hypertension M.D.
mech	Vasodilatation allows for easier blood flow from the heart → decreased blood pressure.	They cause less traffic on the road by making more room for the cars on the roads and in parking lots.
Tox	Reflex tachycardia: Vasodilatation → decreased BP → sympathetic outflow → increased HR	If they are not careful, the HTN M.D.s can decrease the number of cars on the road so much that it "scares" the body. The body likes the roads to be used at a constant level.
Uses	They can all be used for hypertension, even though their use may be limited to hypertensive crisis.	This is the reason they are HTN M.D.s.

Arteriodilators in General

N	Hydralazine, minoxidil, and diazoxide	Things that are used to build larger or faster roads
mech	Dilate arteries and arterioles	They make more room on the roads leading from "Afterload Hill" to the parking lots.

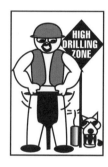

Hydralazine

Tox	Systemic lupus erythematosus because of antihistone antibodies that resolves with discontinuation of the drug	
Uses	Often combined with beta-blockers	
	Congestive heart failure in combination with isosorbide dinitrate	

The High Drilling Zone

There are wolves in the <<high drilling zone>> that may attack the highway workers.

The <<high drilling zone>> can work with the walls that control the vampires and bats.

The <<high drilling zone>> has dynamite in it.

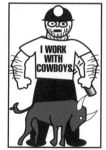

Minoxidil

mech	Metabolized to active metabolites	
Tox	Hirsutism	
	Sodium retention	
Rt	PO only	
Uses	Hair growth in balding	

Miner Building Tunnels for Roads

The miner uses dynamite to build his tunnels.
The miner is very hairy (i.e. beard, etc.).
He also uses steers to build the tunnels.

This is one everyone should know because of the extensive advertising for hair growth. Used for HTN when other drugs don't work.

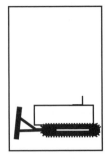

	Diazoxide	**The Bulldozer**
mech	Hyperpolarizes arterial smooth muscle membranes → vasodilation	The bulldozer is used to build roads.
Tox	Inhibits insulin release from pancreas	
Rt	IV and PO	
Uses	Hypertensive emergencies	The bulldozer is heavy equipment for emergencies.

Venodilator: The New York Mets' Parking Lot

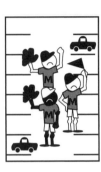

	Trimethaphan*	**Three New York Mets Fans**
N	Trimethaphan	The three New York Mets fans and the parking lot for their stadium.
mech	Direct venodilator	Since there are only three Mets fans there is plenty of room for parking in their lot.
	Also a ganglionic blocker → inhibition of parasympathetic and sympathetics	The three Mets fans stop Nick and Nicky the bear from catching fish from Ganglion Lake.
Tox	Anticholinergic and antisympathetic side effects	¢: Side effects are a result of blockade of both SNS and PNS.
Rt	IV only	
Uses	Only in hypertensive emergencies	Only in horrible traffic, would anyone want to go to a Mets game.

Arterial and Venodilators

Nitrates: Things Road Workers Use to Build Roads and Parking Lots

You can use the picture for these, or you can simply envision the ideal medication for the treatment of angina, and you should be able to arrive at most of the characteristics of the nitrates.

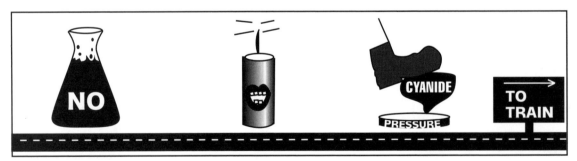

Nitroglycerine	**Isosorbide Dinitrate**	**Sodium Nitroprusside**
N		The road workers use:
Nitroglycerine		Liquid nitroglycerine
Isosorbide dinitrate		Dynamite
Sodium nitroprusside		Pressure mines to build roads and parking lots.
mech	Simulate nitric oxide → increased cGMP → vasodilatation throughout the body:	

*Please also see the chapter on the autonomic nervous system.

	<u>Veno</u>dilation → decreased venous return	These can be used to build <u>parking lots</u> → fewer cars to return to the Phunny Pharm train.
	<u>Arteriolar</u> dilation	They can also be used to build <u>roads</u> to the parking lots.
	Block coronary vasospasm: Subendocardium gets the major share of the benefit, which is the most deprived in the first place.	The road workers can open roads leading to the train, which allows more supplies to get to the train.
$t_{1/2}$	Nitroglycerine—very short ⇒ 2–4'	Nitroglycerine is a liquid and lasts for a shorter time than dynamite.
	Isosorbide <u>dinitrate</u>—longer than nitroglycerine	
Met	Large first-pass elimination by the liver	If the road workers go by the police station,* then they are handcuffed for carrying explosives in public.
Tox	Sodium nitroprusside → thiocyanate and cyanide toxicity	The pressure mine can release cyanide → damage to the Phunny Pharm.
SE's	Reflex sympathetic activity secondary to a fall in blood pressure → reflex tachycardia and splanchnic vasoconstriction.	If the road workers open too many roads, they scare the train and it goes faster.
	Headache secondary to distended meningeal vessels	Dynamite road work at the University causes traffic jams → headaches at the University campus.†
Rt	Nitroglycerine—IV, sublingual, transdermal, PO requires large doses secondary to first pass metabolism by liver.	
	Isosorbide dinitrate—<u>PO</u>	Dynamite has a <u>mouth</u> on it.
	Sodium nitroprusside—<u>IV</u> only	The pressure mine is made of <u>ivory</u>.
Uses	Angina—by increased blood flow to the heart and decreasing preload → less work for the heart.	They all can build larger roads to the heart. They also decrease the number of cars getting on the train by making more room for them in the parking lots.
	Tolerance develops with repeated use and with long-acting preparations secondary to dependence upon a sulfhydryl group depletion. Acetylcysteine can be used to replenish SH groups, or "holidays" from the medication must be taken.	
	Nitroglycerine—used for acute anginal attack	
	Isosorbide dinitrate—prophylaxis of angina and congestive heart failure in combination with hydralazine	
	Sodium nitroprusside—heart failure and aortic valve insufficiency (anytime continuous and immediate preload reduction is needed)	

Ca^{+2} Channel Antagonists: Restaurants Distracting Cows

N	Dihydropyridines ⇒ nifedipine, isradipine, nicardipine, felodipine, amlodipine	The Water/Pie Diner
	Verapamil, diltiazem, bepridil	The restaurant car on the Phunny Pharm train
mech	Blocks Ca^{+2} entry into cells → (≡ smooth musculature) vasodilation	The restaurants distract cows so that they do not close roads.

---

*Rem: The liver is represented by the Phunny Pharm jail and police station throughout <u>The Phunny Pharm</u>.
†Rem: The CNS is represented by the Phunny Pharm University throughout <u>The Phunny Pharm</u>.

Met	All are by the liver.	The Phunny Pharm police can close the restaurants.
SE's	Constipation—worse with verapamil	
Tox	Negative inotropy: Ca^{+2} is needed to uncover myosin binding sites $\Rightarrow$ if there is no $Ca^{+2} \rightarrow$ myosin heads cannot work.	The cows on the Phunny Pharm Train cannot help shovel coal so that the engine will work; therefore, the train gets weaker.
Uses	Hypertension Angina	
R_x/R_x	Cimetidine inhibits calcium channel antagonist metabolism Decrease clearance of digoxin $\rightarrow$ increased digoxin levels.	

Dihydropyridines   The Water/Pie Diner

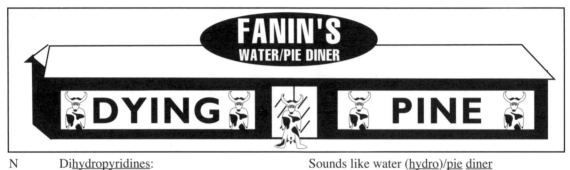

N	Dihydropyridines: They all end in -dipine The first letters spell FANIN: felodipine, amlodipine, nifedipine, isradipine, nicardipine	Sounds like water (hydro)/pie diner Dying pine is written in the window. FANIN's Diner
SE's	Reflex tachycardia $\Rightarrow$ calcium channel blockade $\rightarrow$ vasodilation $\rightarrow \downarrow$ BP $\rightarrow \uparrow$ HR	¢
Tox	Amlodipine is the only one that does not cause negative inotropy.	
Uses	Hypertension	The cows cannot destroy roads while they are in the diner $\rightarrow$ more roads upon which the cars can drive.
	Angina Not used for arrhythmias	The cows in the diner are not allowed on the train.

Other Calcium Channel Antagonists:

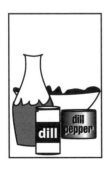

Bepridil, Verapamil, and Diltiazem

N	Bepridil, verapamil, and diltiazem
SE's	Reflex tachycardia not as prominent as with dihydropyridines
Tox	Should not be used in Wolff-Parkinson-White or ventricular tachycardia

Dill Pepper, Vinaigrette, and Dill

(BVD) toppings for a salad $\Rightarrow$ dill pepper (i.e., "pepper dill"), vinaigrette, and dill

	Decrease AV nodal conduction*	The salad decreases the rate of the Phunny Pharm train by distracting the cows, who are driving it.
	Bepridil → torsades de pointes†	
Uses	Also used for supraventricular arrhythmias	
	Class IV antiarrhythmics	Seen also in the chapter on antiarrhythmics
Rₓ/Rₓ	Can cause complete AV nodal blockade with other blockers ⇒ digoxin and β-blockers	

Angiotensin Converting Enzyme Inhibitors: Army Members

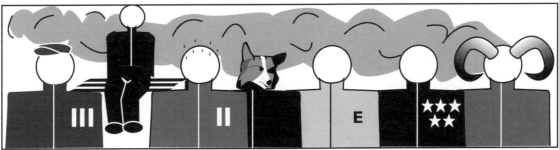

Captopril **Lisinopril** **Enalapril** **Ramipril**
Benazepril **Fosinopril** **Quinapril**

N	All end in -pril	Members of the Army who shoot down the ACE pilot.
	Captopril	The captain of the Army—he wears a cap
	Lisinopril	The lieutenant in the Army—he has lice
	Enalapril	The ensign in the Army
	Ramipril	The recruit to the Army—he is a ram
	Benazepril	The brigadier general—he sits on a bench
	Fosinopril	The foxhole digger—he is a fox
	Quinapril	The five-star general—quin = 5
mech	Vasodilators—Prevent conversion of angiotensin I → angiotensin II. Angiotensin II is a potent vasoconstrictor; therefore, they prevent the formation of the vasoconstrictor.	They shoot down the ACE fighter pilot, whose primary mission is to destroy roads. Therefore, they protect the roads.
	Enalapril is a prodrug that is "activated" to enalaprilat by the liver.	He is beginning to become another active member of the Army (i.e., he will move up in the ranks).
SE's	May increase potassium and creatinine	Can increase the pigs and hurt the showers.
Tox	**Cough,** rash, decreased taste	They cough from the smoke of their tank.
Rt	PO	
Uses	Hypertension and congestive heart failure	
	After a myocardial infarction, → ↓ mortality	
	Prevent renal damage in diabetics	

*This may also be seen as the desired effect of the medications.
†Torsades de pointes is a serious ventricular arrhythmia.

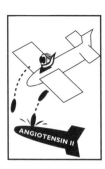

Losartan

N   Losartan

mech   Angiotensin II receptor inhibitor →
        prevents angiotensin II from →
        vasoconstriction and production of
        aldosterone → vasodilation and
        decreases blood pressure

SE's $$Cost$$; although not as expensive
        as captopril
        No cough
        Can increase K

Rt   PO*

The <u>Lost</u> <u>Airman</u>

The Lost Airman on the Army's side
He flies his plane and shoots the
    <<angiotensin II>> bombs as
    they fall onto the road → prevents
    them from hitting the ground →
    saves the roads from destruction.
It costs a lot of money to be able to
    blow up bombs as they fall.
There is no smoke up in the air.
Can increase the number of pigs

---

*Please note: This is the only thing in <u>The Phunny Pharm</u> that flies but cannot be taken in aerosolized form or does not exist in gas form.

Diuretics—Cattle Drive Trail

The kidney retains needed compounds and discards waste products for the body. It accomplishes this by "filtering" the blood through the glomerulus and then reclaiming the items the body needs. This can be likened to pushing fluid through a filter, with the pressure applied to the fluid similar to the blood pressure at the glomerulus. After the filtrate passes through the glomerulus, it passes through a "column" wherein transport mechanisms reclaim the needed items. The urine ultimately contains only waste products, ions, and water that must be present to keep the compounds in solution.

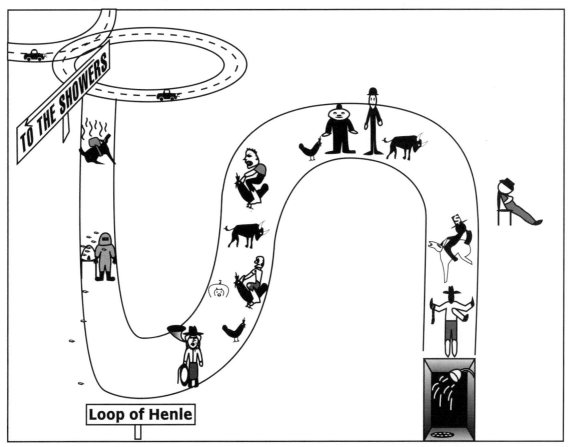

Picture Key

This is a picture of an "animal drive" in which cowboys are trying to steal animals from the body. On this trail, the cowboys (i.e., the diuretics) drive the animals to the end of the trail where showers await them, while the rustlers (i.e., the renal transport mechanisms) attempt to steal the animals back for the body.

The toilet ⇒ the final destination of the urine

Glomerulus ⇒ where blood is filtered
Tubular system of the nephron
Renal transport mechanisms within the nephron

The shower at the end of the trail ⇒ the place to which the cowboys are trying to take the animals.
The mouth of the trail to the cowboys' shower
Trail leading to the cowboys' shower
The rustlers who wait for the animals to come down the trail, and steal them back for The Phunny Pharm

Diuretics

Uses: Hypertension and congestive heart failure

The cowboys herding the animals toward their
    shower
Cowboys make more room on the streets by
    taking the animals and flies to their shower.

Renal Transport Mechanisms

It is a good idea to review renal transport mechanisms. Although it would be great if you could know
all of these pumps, transporters, and channels and the areas in the nephron in which these work, I could never
keep them straight. Therefore, I have narrowed the number of transport mechanisms to the bare minimum
needed to begin to understand the diuretics.

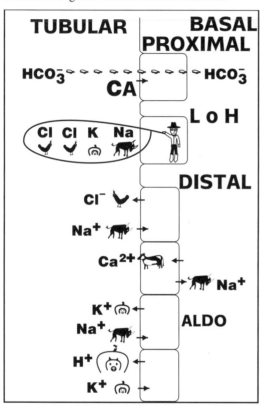

1. Bicarbonate moves
   across the tubular cells
   using carbonic
   anhydrase (CA).

   Carbonic anhydrase dries
   the bee's wings so
   they can fly out of the
   hives and back into
   the body.

2. In the ascending loop of
   Henle (LoH), a
   cotransporter moves
   Na/K/2Cl into the
   tubular cells.

   This is the main place on
   the trail where the
   rustlers steal the
   animals back from the
   cowboys.

3. The distal convoluted
   tubule has a couple of
   transporters that are
   important:

   At the end of the trail,
   the rustlers hide and
   make final adjustments
   on the animals the
   Phunny Pharm needs.

   Na/Ca exchanger on the
   basolateral side

   One trades steers for
   cows.

   Na/K exchanger on tubular
   side (aldosterone →
   retention of Na and loss
   of K)

   One trades steers for
   pigs.

   K/H exchanger on tubular
   side

   One trades pigs for hogs.

Side Effects

If the above mechanisms and the diuretics' location of action can be remembered, the usual side effects
of diuretics can be deduced.

Hypokalemia accompanies metabolic alkalosis. Any
    decrease in K^+ presented to the distal convoluted
    tubule will result in a decrease in H^+ in the body as
    the kidney attempts to retain K^+.

In the picture, hogs are H^+ ions and pigs are
    potassium. Because these are the same type of
    animal, they stay together. Also note that this
    happens by the K/H exchanger.

Hypercalcemia or hypocalcemia: An increase in the Na^+
    within the distal convoluted tubule cells results in loss
    of Ca as Na^+ is traded for Ca → hypocalcemia. But, if
    the Na^+/Cl cotransporter is blocked at the tubular side
    of the cells, there is no Na^+ to be traded for the Ca
    within the tubular cells and → hypercalcemia.

Many of the diuretics are transported into the tubule via a
    carrier competing with organic acids such as uric acid
    and penicillins. Therefore, another side effect can
    result from increases in uric acid and manifest as
    gout or prolongation of penicillin half-life.

Drugs excreted via this mechanism:
    Penicillin
    Acetaminophen
    Thiazides

Osmotic Diuretics

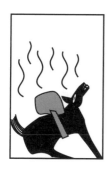

Mannit**ol**

mech	Filtered at the glomerulus and not reabsorbed
Tox	Inhibits reabsorption of $\underline{H_2O}$, but has no effect on solutes → Hypernatremia
Uses	Increases urine volume drastically
	<u>Cerebral</u> edema

Dirty <u>Ol' Mule</u>

Exits the road, but the cowboys do not want to rescue the mule, so it does not reenter the body

<u>Flies</u> follow it just like any animal to the cowboys' hideout.

The mule does not care what the steers do, so they become abundant compared to the flies.

Because it is such a dirty ol' mule, it attracts a lot of flies.

Employed by the Phunny Pharm <u>University</u>* to rid it of its flies

Carbonic Anhydrase Inhibitors

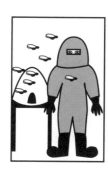

Acetaz**ol**amide

mech	Inhibits carbonic anhydrase, which prevents formation of CO_2 from HCO_3^-. Therefore, there is loss of $NaHCO_3$.
Tox	Loss of HCO_3^- → metabolic acidosis
Uses	<u>Glau</u>coma

Ace the Ol' Beekeeper

Ace puts them in their boxes so they will make honey for the cowboys, and prevents them from flying† out of the trail. Thus, the bees cannot reenter the body.

This should be easy, but can also be remembered by "Ace is an acidic ol' feller."

The bees' honey is sticky, like <u>glue</u>.

Loop Diuretics In General

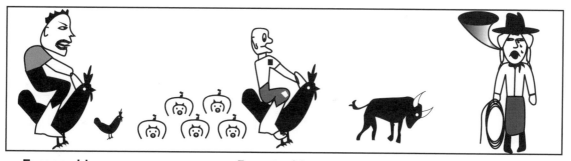

Furosemide　　　　**Bumetanide**　　　　**Ethacrynic Acid**

N	Loop diuretics:

<u>Furosemide</u>
<u>Bumetan</u>ide
<u>Ethacry</u>nic acid

mech	Inhibit the Na/K/2Cl cotransporter in the ascending limb of the <u>loop</u> of Henle.

These cowboys who are herding the animals toward their shower rope the rustlers with a <u>loop</u> of rope to keep them from stealing the animals back.

<u>Furious</u> <u>Mike</u>
The ol' <u>bum</u> who likes to <u>ride</u>
<u>Ethyl</u> the <u>crying</u> cowgirl

Rope the rustler who is trying to steal the steers, pigs, and chickens with a <u>loop</u>.

---

*Rem: The nervous system is represented by the University.

†Rem: Anything that can fly represents the gaseous form of the compound.

$t_{1/2}$	Furosemide is short → abrupt onset of diuresis.	He's furious, so he's very fast.
	Bumetanide is longer than furosemide.	The bum is not as mad as Furious Mike.
Tox	<u>Ototoxicity</u>, especially ethacrynic acid	These cowboys have shot too many guns ⇒ <u>can't hear</u>. Ethyl cries enough for your ears to hurt.
	Hypokalemia	Because they have so many steers by the time they get to the end of the trail, they will trade the rustlers for pigs and cows → a depletion of pigs and cows in the Phunny Pharm.
	Hypocalcemia	
Uses	Hypertension	They remove animals from the Phunny Pharm roads → makes more room on the roads and makes it easier for the Phunny Pharm train to run.
	Heart failure	
	Fluid overload	They are also used when there is just too many things on the Phunny Pharm Roads.

Thiazide Diuretics

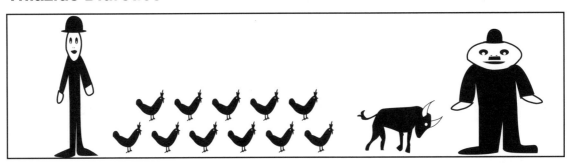

Chlorothiazide   **Hydrochlorothiazide**

N	Chlorothiazide	Laurel
	Hydrochlorothiazide	Hardy
mech	Inhibit the Na/Cl cotransporter in the distal tubule; works from the tubular side	Sit on the steers and the chickens so that the rustlers cannot take the animals back
	Secreted into tubule by organic acid carrier*	
	Hydrochlorothiazide is 10x as potent as chlorothiazide.	Hardy is 10x as big as Laurel.
Tox	Hypokalemia as sodium is retained in exchange for potassium.	The rustlers realize that they don't have enough steers, so they trade them for the pigs at the end of the trail.
	Kidney stones	
	Hypercalcemia	They hate cows, so they do not let the rustlers trade them for their steers.
	Hyperuricemia	They get gout because they are so big.
Uses	Hypertension	They remove animals and flies from the roads, making more room on the Phunny Pharm roads.

---

*Note: They will not work in Renal Insufficiency because they must be excreted into the tubule to work.

Aldosterone Antagonists: Potassium Sparing

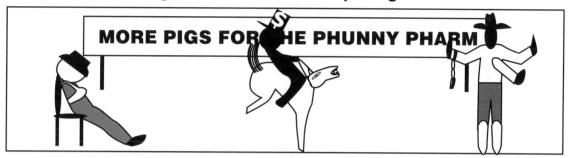

	Spironolactone	**Amiloride**	**Triamterene**
N	Their first letters spell <u>SAT</u>: Spironolac<u>tone</u> <u>A</u>miloride <u>T</u>riam<u>t</u>erine	Cowboys who <u>SAT</u> at the end of the trail, and guard the animals from the rustlers. In essence, they balance out the animals that they take to the shower. A <u>spy</u> who sits <u>alone</u> A <u>millionaire</u> who likes to <u>ride</u> <u>Three</u>-armed cowboy <u>steers</u> the steers	
mech	Block an aldosterone-dependent Na/K exchange in distal convoluted tubule → retention of K in the body and Na loss in the urine. Spironolactone competitively antagonizes aldosterone ⇒ it must work from the basolateral side of the cells. Amiloride and triamterine directly inhibit the Na transporter from the tubular side.	These cowboys keep the rustlers from trading pigs for steers, so the rustlers have to hold on to their pigs → the Phunny Pharm to have more pigs. The spy prevents pigs from being traded, by infiltrating into the rustler network as a spy (i.e., he works on the inside). Because the millionaire and three-armed cowboy are not experienced at covert operations like the spy, they physically stop the steer/pig trade.	
Met	Triamterine ⇒ liver clearance is high	The three-armed cowboy gets arrested* because he causes trouble in town.	
Tox	Hyperkalemia Spironolactone has occasional estrogen-like effects ⇒ gynecomastia and amenorrhea	The rustlers hold on to all of the pigs that they have → too many pigs in the Phunny Pharm. The <u>spy</u> occasionally has to dress like a lady and therefore must wear a <u>bra.</u>	
Uses	Prevent the loss of K Often used in conjunction with loop diuretics for synergism or to decrease loss of K.	As above They are good friends with Furious Mike and the bum who likes to ride.	

*Rem: The Phunny Pharm jail and police station represent the liver throughout <u>The Phunny Pharm</u>.

Cardiac Inotropes—StrongerTrain

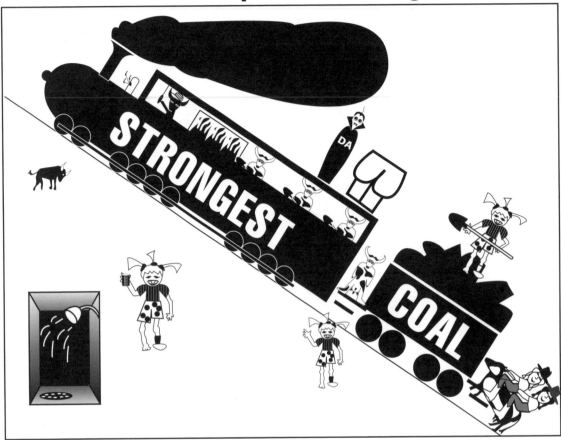

Picture Key

In this chapter, we focus on the Phunny Pharm train. Here we find ways to make the train, which represents the heart, stronger. This is very important in patients who have congestive heart failure. Other drugs are usually used with the inotropes to make pumping easier.

<u>Na</u> is the main ion responsible for the depolarization of the <u>myocardium</u>.

<u>Ca</u> must be present to open binding sites for the myosin heads and thereby allow a <u>contraction</u>.

<u>Inotropy</u>, which is usually a result of increased intracellular Ca

The <u>steers</u> are the engineers and are responsible for the speed of the <u>train</u>.

<u>Cows</u> in the engine are responsible for shoveling coal into the fire so the train will have <u>energy</u>.

<u>Stronger engines</u>—they are stronger when there are more cows to shovel the coal.

Inotropic Agents in General

N   <u>Digitalis</u>
      <u>Digoxin</u>
      <u>Digitoxin</u>
      <u>Amrinone</u>
      <u>Dobutamine</u>
      <u>Dopamine</u>

<u>Ditzy Alice</u>
    <u>Dig in</u> ditzy Alice
    More <u>toxic</u> than digoxin
<u>Amy riding one</u>
<u>Dracula's</u> butt is a <u>mean</u> one
<u>Dopey</u> <u>Dean</u> the <u>mean</u> vampire

mech   All increase intracellular Ca → more open myosin binding sites → increased cardiac contractility → increased cardiac output

All of the things that increase the strength of the engines do so by increasing the number of cows to shovel coal into the fire.

Digitalis (Digoxin, Digitoxin)   # Ditzy Alice

Mechanism of Action

It is very important to understand the following mechanism. The end result is an increase in intracellular Ca → increased contractility. In the Phunny Pharm, Ditzy Alice doesn't let cows out of the engine → more cows to shovel coal on the fire and therefore the train is stronger.

In the Normal Cardiac Cell
A Na/K ATP-dependent pump moves Na out of the cell and K into the cell.
There is also a 4Na/Ca exchanger that utilizes the electrochemical gradient of Na to move Ca out of the cell as Na moves into the cell.

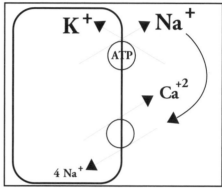

Digitalis Inotropic Efect
Digitalis binds competitively with K and inhibits the Na/K ATP-dependent pump → intracellular Na to increase → a smaller electrochemical gradient.
The smaller drive for Na to enter the cell decreases the amount of Ca removed from the cell, and intracellular Ca increases within the sarcoplasma reticulum.
Increased Ca → increased Ca binding of troponin during contraction → open myosin binding sites → increased contractility.

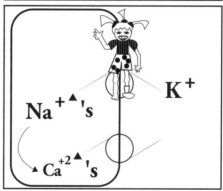

Digitalis Electrophysiologic Effects
Indirect Effect (seen at therapeutic levels):
Increase sensitivity of the heart to vagal stimulation → decreased SA node depolarizations and conduction through the AV node.
Direct (seen at toxic levels):
Higher intracellular Ca → predisposition for "after depolarizations"

Ditzy Alice helps the three musketeer cubs* slow down the train, while she makes it stronger.

When Ditzy Alice is around too much, there gets to be too many cows in the engine and they cannot coordinate themselves to run the engine.

Low extracellular K → increased risk of hypokalemic arrhythmias
Almost any arrhythmia can occur, especially AV block; also premature ventricular contractions, ventricular tachycardia, and fibrillation

---

*Rem: The three musketeers cubs' actions represent a stimulation of muscarinic receptors (i.e., parasympathetic) throughout the Phunny Pharm.

Digitalis in General

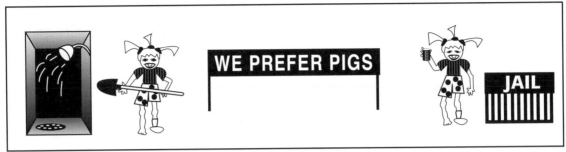

	Digoxin	**Digitoxin**
N	There are two types of digitalis: Digoxin Digitoxin	Dig in ditzy Alice More toxic ditzy Alice
mech	Other effects: Diureses secondary to inotropy Arterio- and venodilation secondary to decreased sympathetic drive. No change in myocardial oxygen demands	¢: Increased inotropy → increased pressure at the kidney ¢: Vasodilation from decreased sympathetic drive counterbalances increased contractility of the heart.
Met	Renal Digitoxin hepatic	Dig in can be seen on her way to the showers.
$t_{1/2}$	Digoxin is shorter than digitoxin	Since digitoxin is more toxic, she gets put in jail. The word "digoxin" is smaller than "digitoxin."
Tox	Low therapeutic index Hypokalemia → increased toxicity because K competes with digitalis for binding to the Na/K exchanger ⟹ with less K, there is more digoxin effect. GI ⟹ Nausea/vomitting CNS ⟹ fatigue, hallucinations Visual ⟹ objects look yellow	¢: Digitalis competes for binding with K. If there is low K, then there will be a larger effect by digitalis. Ditzy Alice is tired after making the cows remain on the train, and her black and white television begins to take on colors.
Rt	Digoxin—PO and IV Digitoxin—PO only	
Uses	Congestive heart failure ⟹ increases inotropy, diuresis, decreased heart rate, and venodilation. Therefore → increased inotropy without changing O_2 demand. Supraventricular arrhythmias—decrease the ventricular response to atrial depolarizations	Ditzy Alice can be used when traffic on the Phunny Pharm roads is too congested.
R_x/R_x	Toxicity increased by sympathomimetics, Ca, Mg, hypokalemia. Digoxin clearance decreased by quinidine, verapamil, amiodarone, flecainide, and propafenone.	

Other Inotropic Agents in General

mech Increase cAMP → increased Ca entry during contraction

They all camp on top of the engine and make more cows dump coal on the fire.

Uses Congestive heart failure

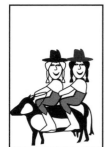

Amrinone and Milrinone

N Amrinone
  Milrinone
mech Phosphodiesterase inhibitors → increased cAMP→ increased Ca entry during contraction → increased contractility
Tox Hepatotoxicity
  Thrombocytopenia

Amy and Milly Riding One

Amy riding one, (i.e., a cow)
Milly riding one
They camp on a cow and ride her into the engine so she can shovel more coal → a stronger engine

They ride their cow over the Phunny Pharm jail and Corvettes*

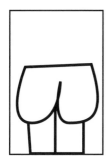

Dobutamine†

mech β₁-receptor agonist → increased cAMP → increased Ca entry during contraction → increased contractility

Also agonist for α and β₂ but → no net change in peripheral vascular resistance.
Rt IV only

Dracula's Butt Is a Mean One

Dracula's mean butt scares the vampires to camp out. These vampires make the cows work harder → stronger Phunny Pharm train.
¢: The effects balance each other out since α → vasoconstriction, and β₂ → vasodilation

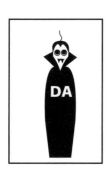

Dopamine

mech Precursor of norepinephrine and epinephrine
  Low doses → stimulation of dopaminergic receptors in renal arteries → vasodilation
  Higher doses → β₁-receptor agonism → increased cardiac contractility
  Also → direct release of norepinephrine
  Higher doses → α₁-receptor agonism → vasoconstriction.
Uses At low doses, diuresis in CHF and renal failure Hypotension

Dopey Dean the Mean Vampire

Scares other vampires into making the train stronger.
Scares cowboys to speed up their drive to the Phunny Pharm shower.

At high doses, he scares antelope into closing roads.
¢: from mechanism

---

*Rem: The liver and platelets are represented by the Phunny Pharm jail and Corvettes throughout The Phunny Pharm.
†Please also see dobutamine and dopamine in the ANS chapter on sympathomimetics for more details.

Antiarrhythmics—Train Cars Interfering with the Engineers of the Train

Although there are many antiarrhythmics in use, it is important to remember that only beta blockers and Ca^{+2} channel blockers have been shown to prolong life.

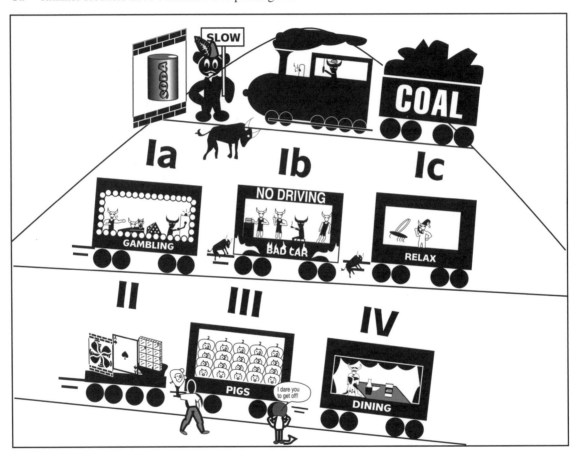

Picture Key

This picture focuses upon the function of the Phunny Pharm train engines, and the coordination of their movement up "Pressure Hill."

Heart — The train

Na$^+$ — Steers—the engineers of the train

Ca^{+2} — Cows—the animals responsible for putting coal into the fire so that the engine will pull

K$^+$ — Pigs

Antiarrythmics — Train cars behind the train's engines that interfere with the normal function of the engines.

Ions Responsible for Action Potentials and Picture Key

Action potentials occur in all cardiac cells and are either the sole purpose of the cell, as in the conduction system, or facilitate the action of the cell, as in the myocardial cells. The action potential is initiated in cells of the nodes, it is conducted and propagated through Purkinje cells, and finally causes contraction as it reaches myocardial cells. This action potential is divided into five phases and can be seen in the following picture:

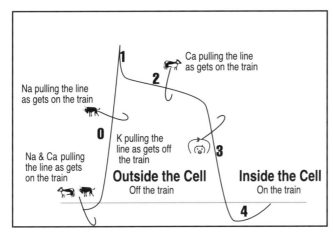

The ions responsible for each phase of the action potential, if you can visualize the line of the action potential as the cell membrane. The more positive side of the line is the inside of the cell and the more negative side, the outside. The ionic movements in each phase of the action potential are hooks that "pull" the line with them as they move across the membrane. For the Phunny Pharm, the animals can also be visualized pulling the action potential.

Phase 0—Na^+ *enters* via <u>fast channels</u>, and there is a rapid upstroke of the action potential.

Phase I—The action potential "overshoots" the peak.

Phase II—Ca^{+2} *enters* the cell via <u>slow channels</u>, maintaining the potential at a plateau.

Phase III—K^+ *exits* cell and causes a rapid repolarization.

Phase IV—Ca^{+2} and Na^+ *enter* the cell to cause slow depolarization (i.e., decay) towards threshold. When the depolarization reaches threshold, phase 0 begins again.

<u>Steers quickly</u> get on the train. In myocardial cells, when there are enough of them in the engine, they begin to drive the train up Pressure Hill.

<u>Cows slowly</u> get on the train. In myocardial cells, they are picked up along the track and put coal on the fire, so the engine can pull itself up Pressure Hill.

<u>Pigs</u> get out of the train. In myocardial cells, as pigs get out, the engines quit working and the train is pulled back to the bottom of Pressure Hill.

<u>Cows</u> and <u>steers</u> slowly begin to get back on the train at the bottom of the hill. When there is enough of them on board, the steers begin to get on quicker (i.e., go to phase 0).

Types of Depolarizations (= Action Potential)

Take note that there are essentially two ions that are responsible for depolarization, Na^+ and Ca^{+2}. Each ion uses its own channel to enter the cell; Na^+ passes through fast channels, and Ca^{+2} uses slow channels. Because of this, there can be two types of action potentials in the cells, depending upon which channels are present. If both types of channels are present, a fast response action potential is produced, whereas a slow response action potential is produced when Na^+ channels are not present. Notice also that the slow response action potential is essentially the fast response action potential without the influence of the fast Na^+ channels of phase 0.

<u>Fast response fibers</u>: Na^+ channels are present.
    Fast response is found in:
        Myocardial fibers of atria and ventricles
        Purkinje fibers ⇒ specialized conducting fibers

<u>Slow response</u>: No fast response Na^+ channels are present; therefore, action potential is dependent only on slow Ca^{+2} channels.
    Slow response is found in:
      SA node
      AV node

Rhythms and Arrhythmias

The timing of the contraction of the heart is essential for proper function of the pump and when it fails, the results can be disastrous. The arrhythmias are difficult to learn, and at this point it is only important to understand the very basics. You will learn to recognize specific rhythms on the wards.

Sinus rhythm ⇒ Any rhythm originating from the <u>sinus</u> node

Junctional rhythm ⇒ Any rhythm originating from the AV node

Flutter ⇒ Rapid discharge of action potentials from a cell that takes over pacemaking capacity

Fibrillation ⇒ Many different cells discharging with no synchronicity

Antiarrhythmics in General

N	Class Ia—Na^+ channel blockers	The gambling car
	Class Ib—Na^+ channel blockers	The "<u>b</u>ad" car
	Class Ic—Na^+ channel blockers	The relaxation car
	Class II—β-adrenergic blockers	The car with walls that will stop the train
	Class III—K^+ channel blockers	The car where all of the pigs go
	Class IV—Ca^{+2} channel blockers	The restaurant car
	Others:	
	Adenosine	A musketeer bear cub holding a sign = "slow down"
	<u>Sotolol</u>	A <u>tall</u> <u>so</u>da <u>wall</u>
Tox	Mainly due to proarrhythmic action	
	Negative inotropy	
Uses	Used for arrhythmias, but only β-adrenergic blockers and calcium channel blockers have been shown to prolong life.	
R_x/R_x	Antiarrhythmics have a cumulative effect on the action potential.	

<u>Class I Antiarrhythmics</u>

Class Ia in General   The Gambling Car

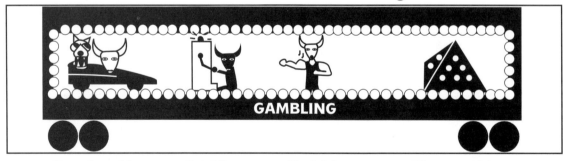

	Procainamide Quinidine	**Moricizine Disopyramide**
N	<u>Class Ia antiarrhythmics:</u>	The gambling car that distracts the steers with the thought "<u>pros win more</u> in <u>dice</u>."*
	<u>Procaina</u>mide	<u>Pros can</u> bet on auto racing.
	<u>Quini</u>dine	<u>Win dimes</u> at the slot machines.
	<u>Mor</u>icizine	<u>More easy to sing</u>
	<u>Dis</u>opyramide	<u>Dice</u> in the shape of <u>pyramids</u>
mech	Use-dependent blockade of fast Na^+ channels by binding the Na^+ channels in the open state → slower conduction of AP.	The steers see the gambling sign and would rather play dice than go into the train's engine through the fast channels.

*Note: These are the first part of each drug name.

	Also decreases slope of phase IV → decreased automaticity	Because steers do not enter the engines, the engine does not move as much as it would if there were more steers in the engine. Steers are also not getting on train during phase IV.
	Prolong conduction time and refractoriness In addition, class Ia also exhibits vagolytic effects, especially at the AV node → <u>increased</u> conduction through the node.	
Met	Procainamide undergoes N-acetyl transferase in liver → production of N-acetyl procainamide (<u>NAPA</u>)	They bet upon the <u>NAPA</u> race car.
	Procainamide ⇒ renal and heart failure → decreased clearance.	
	Quinidine ⇒ hepatic P-450 hydroxylation	
	Disopyramide ⇒ 50% renal	
Cells affected	<u>Mainly</u> atrial and ventricular muscle	¢: These are the tissues that are dominated by the Na channels.
Tox	Hypotension	
	Torsade de Pointes	The steers lose so much that they get their horns (i.e., points) tied in a knot.
	Procainamide → <u>lupus</u>-like syndrome, bone marrow suppression	The race car is up against the <u>wolves</u>* who are driving a car.
	Quinidine → hypotension from alpha-adrenergic blockade.	Win dimes to keep antelope from blocking the roads → vasodilation.
	Cinchonism	It is a cinch to win on these slot machines.
Rt	All IV except disopyramide ⇒ only PO	
Uses	Arrhythmias not originating in a node	¢: No effect at the nodes.
	In atrial arrhythmias, the AV node should be blocked prior to use; since vagolytic effects can → increased ventricular response to atrial fibrillation/flutter.	¢
R$_x$/R$_x$	P-450 inducers → increased clearance of quinidine	
	P-450 inhibitors → decreased clearance of quinidine; especially cimetidine and amiodarone	

Class Ib in General   The "<u>B</u>ad" Car

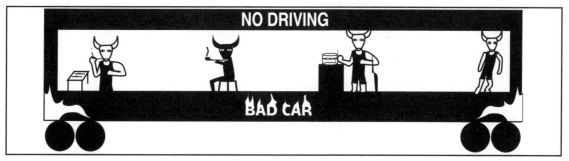

	Lidocaine Tocainide	**Mexiletine Phenytoin**
N	Class Ib antiarrhythmics:	Things in this car are related to drugs and therefore distract the steers.
	<u>Lidocaine</u>	<u>Light</u> up some co<u>caine</u>.
	<u>To</u>cainide—essentially oral lidocaine	<u>To</u>ke up some marijuana.

*Rem: Lupus means wolf throughout <u>The Phunny Pharm</u>.

	Mexiletine	Steers <u>mix a little</u> drink.
	Phenytoin	When the steers have taken the drugs, they walk <u>funny</u> with their <u>toes in</u>.*
mech	Na$^+$ channel blockade in open and closed state.	¢: All class I block Na channel.
	Decrease slope of phase IV; particularly in abnormal automatic cells → suppression of aberrant pacemakers.	They distract the steers and get them so "high" that they do not want to drive the engine out of the station.
	Shorten APD	
Cells affected	Usually only fast channel tissues: Atrial and ventricular muscle and His-Purkinje	¢: These are the tissues dominated by the Na channels.
	Also ischemic tissue	
Met	Lidocaine ≈ 100% <u>hepatic</u> ⇒ large first-pass metabolism prevents PO administration.	The <u>cops</u>† are extremely against smoking crack.
Tox	Lidocaine ⇒ somnolence, confusion	
	Tocainide ⇒ <u>granulocytosis</u>	When the steers do toke up some marijuana, they hallucinate ⇒ they have <u>grand 'ol sights</u>.
Rt	Lidocaine ⇒ IV	
	Tocainide, mexiletine ⇒ PO	
Uses	Wide range of ventricular arrhythmias only ⇒ no supraventricular arrhythmias.	
	Abolish delayed afterpotentials owing to digitalis toxicity.	
	Tocainide ⇒ limited due to granulocytosis	Get scared when they hallucinate (have grand ol' sights); therefore it is not used much.

Class Ic in General   The Relaxation Car

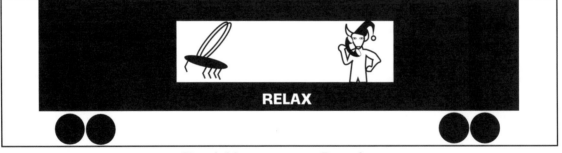

	Flecainide	**Propafenone**
N	Class Ic antiarrhythmics: Flecainide Propafenone	A car in which the steers relax: <u>Fleas can hide</u> on the steers. <u>Pro</u> steers <u>can phone home</u>.
mech	Decrease slope of phase 0.	
	Slightly increase action potential duration and effective refractory period.	
	Propafenone — also has weak β-blocking properties	The pro steers can phone home and tell the vampires and bats not to scare the Phunny Pharm.
Tox	Negative inotropy	
Uses	Last choice in life-threatening arrhythmias	

---

*Phenytoin is also seen in the CNS chapter.
†Rem: Hepatic metabolism is symbolized by policemen and jails throughout <u>The Phunny Pharm</u>.

Class II in General   The Car with Walls that Stop the Train

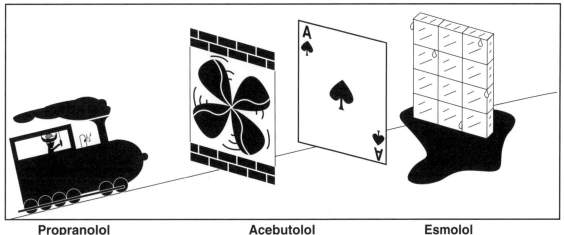

	Propranolol	**Acebutolol**	**Esmolol**
N	Class II in general:		The car with walls that stop the train:

N — Class II in general:
    Propran<u>olol</u>
    Acebut<u>olol</u>
    Esm<u>olol</u>

The car with walls that stop the train:
    <u>Prop</u>eller <u>wall</u>
    <u>Ace</u> wall
    <u>Es</u>kimo wall

mech — β-adrenergic blockade → decreased slope of phase IV in SA and AV nodes, and → prolongation of AV nodal conduction.

They all prevent bats and vampires from getting to the train, such that they slow it down.

Cells affected — Only slow response fibers that respond to adrenergic innervation

¢: Only the cells at the nodes will respond to the walls.

t_{1/2} — Esmolol is a very short acting β-blocker.

The eskimo ice wall melts rapidly.

Tox — Heart failure, asthma exacerbation, and should be used with caution in diabetics

¢: Because of β-blockade

Uses — Supraventricular arrhythmias to convert to sinus rhythm or to slow ventricular response to atrial fibrillation or flutter

Reentry with the AV node as one limb of the pathway

¢: Will slow the arm of the pathway in the node.

Class III in General   Car Where Pigs Go

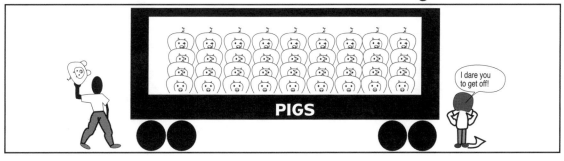

	Bretylium Tosylate	**Amiodarone**

N — Class III antiarrhythmics:

The car where the pigs go, instead of getting off the train. Two people keep the pigs from getting off:

    Bretylium <u>tos</u>ylate

<u>Bret toss</u>es the pigs back onto the train if they get off.

    <u>Ami</u>odarone

<u>Amy dares</u> the pigs to get off of the train.

mech	Blockade of K⁺ channels	Keep pigs from getting off the train.
	Prolong action potential duration and effective refractory prreiod.	¢: K can't repolarize membrane if its channels are blocked. In the Phunny Pharm, the pigs can't pull the line back down.
	Bretylium tosylate → initially causes a release of norepinephrine, and then prevents further release of norepinephrine.	At first, Bret uses a norepi cross to scare the antelope and vampires as well as the pigs, but then he gets tired and prevents others from getting scared by the cross.
Cells affected	Purkinje system and ventricular muscle cells	
$t_{1/2}$	Amiodarone for 20 to 100 days	Amy can dare them for a long time.
Tox	Bretylium tosylate ⇒ hypotension	
	Amiodarone ⇒ many, including:	
	Hyper or hypothyroidism	Amy has big thighs.
	Pulmonary fibrosis	Amy can ruin the Phunny Pharm airport, she is stepping on a lung tube.
Uses	Ventricular fibrillation or sustained tachycardia	
	Supraventricular arrhythmias in low dose	

Class IV in General   The Restaurant Car

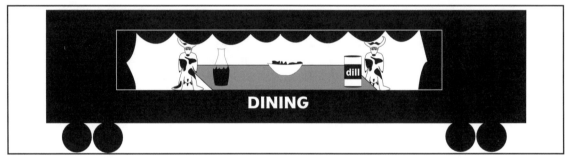

	Verapamil	Diltiazem
N	Class IV antiarrhythmics:	The restaurant car with things that can be put on the salad that the cows will eat.
	Verapamil	Vinaigrette salad dressing
	Diltiazem	Dill to be used on the salads.
mech	Ca⁺² channel blockers	The restaurant car distracts the fat cows so that they do not get into the engine.
	Increase conduction time and "refractoriness" of slow channel cells	The cows get fatter so they can't move as fast. They also have to digest their food before the cows can help with another trip up Pressure Hill; therefore, they increase "refractoriness."
Cells affected	Do not affect cells with fast response fibers; therefore only works at the SA and AV nodes	¢: The primary ion affecting the fast response cells is Na⁺, and these are Ca⁺² channel blockers.
Tox	Hypotension	
	Cannot use in atrial fibrillation in Wolff-Parkinson-White syndrome, because may increase ventricular response	
Uses	Slow the response of the ventricle to atrial fibrillation/flutter	
	Only work on slow channel tissues, therefore only for supraventricular arrhythmias	¢: Ca channel antagonists work best at the nodes.
R_x/R_x	With β-blockers, may cause arrhythmias.	¢: They both work at nodes.

Additional Antiarrhythmics

Adenosine

N   Adeno<u>sine</u>

mech   Resembles actions of acetylcholine actions at the AV node

$t_{1/2}$ Very short—seconds

Tox   Dyspnea

Rt   IV bolus

Uses   Paroxysmal supraventricular tachyarrhythmias

A Musketeer Holding a <u>Sign</u>

A musketeer* bear cub holding a <u>sign</u> that reads "slow down."

The sign slows down the train at the AV node.

The musketeer can't hold the heavy sign for long.

Short of breath because of the heavy sign

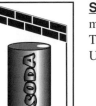

Sotalol

mech   β-blockade activity

Tox   Prolongs QT → torsade de pointes

Uses   Prevention of ventricular tachycardia

A Tall <u>Soda</u> <u>Wall</u>

A tall soda wall slows down the train.

---

*Rem: The three musketeer bear cubs represent the effect of parasympathetic stimulation of muscarinic cholinergic receptors throughout <u>The Phunny Pharm</u>.

Antihyperlipidemics—Fighting Crime

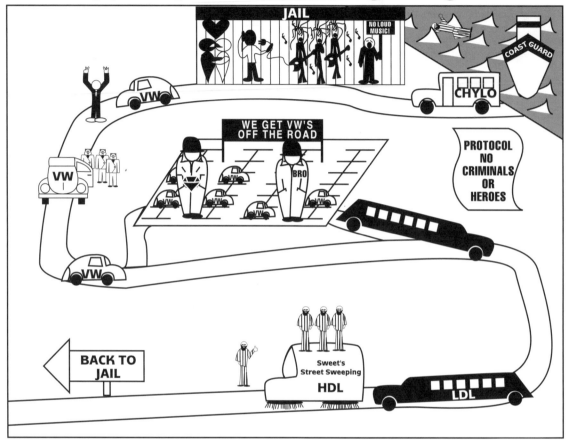

Picture Key

The picture for lipid metabolism and manipulation takes us to the part of the Phunny Pharm where crime is fought. The criminals are, of course, the mean, bad lipoproteins (LDL); the drugs are the people and things responsible for stopping the movement of the criminals; and the good lipoproteins (HDL) are the street sweepers. The sweepers are driven by a reformed criminal who is responsible for cleaning the streets and delivering criminals back to the jail.

Liver	Jail
Gastrointestinal tract	The Phunny Pharm ocean
HMG-CoA reductase	Mean Heavy Metal Group in the jail
<u>C</u>holesterol and <u>t</u>riglycerides:	The bad guys
Both can be ingested in the diet or made in the liver and are virtually insoluble in water.	
<u>C</u>holesterol:	The <u>c</u>riminals
Production of bile, bile acids, and membranes	
<u>T</u>riglyceride (TG):	The <u>tri</u>o of gangsters
Three fatty acids hooked to a glycerol backbone	
The main source of fatty acids for muscle and adipocytes	

Lipoproteins
  Chylomicrons:
    Mainly TGs and small cholesterol
  VLDL:
    TGs and cholesterol.
  LDL:
    Mainly cholesterol
  HDL:
    Mainly cholesterol

Automobiles in which bad guys ride:
A bus carrying bad guys from the border to the jail before they can enter the country
Volkswagen: When the bad guys first get on the street, a VW is all they can afford.
A limo: After the criminals are on the street for a while, they can afford a limo.
The hero: A reformed criminal who picks up criminals from the body and takes them back to the jail. She drives a street sweeper because she "cleans up the city."

Introduction to Lipid Metabolism and Picture Key

The movement of the criminals is analogous to the movement of cholesterol and triglyceride throughout the body. To review quickly:

Distribution of Lipids to the Body

1. Cholesterol and triglycerides (TGs) are placed into chylomicrons by the intestinal epithelium and released into the blood.
2. Liver takes up the chylomicrons, packages TGs and cholesterol into very low density lipoproteins (VLDL), and releases them into the blood.

3. VLDL circulates throughout the body, TGs are removed, the cholesterol becomes more concentrated, and the lipoproteins are converted to LDLs.

4. LDLs distribute cholesterol throughout the body to cells as well as back to the liver.

Synthesis of Cholesterol

1. Cholesterol is made in all cells of the body, but mainly by the liver, with the limiting enzyme being HMG-CoA reductase.

Removal of Lipids from the Body

1. HDLs remove cholesterol.

2. Cholesterol is secreted into the intestine as bile acids.

Bad Guy Entrance into the Phunny Pharm

1. A bus carries the criminals and the trios of gangsters from the border of the Phunny Pharm onto the road.
2. The jail takes the bus, processes the new arrivals to the Phunny Pharm, puts the criminals and the trios of gangsters in a Volkswagon, and sends them down the road.
3. The VW is driven around the Phunny Pharm. As some trios of gangsters get out of the car, the VW criminal concentration increases. When criminals remain and only a few trios of gangsters, they pull into the used car dealer and trade in their VW for a limousine. At this point, they have accumulated the wealth to afford this transaction.
4. The limo is driven throughout the body and lets criminals out along the way. The jail can also take the limos off of the street.

Criminals Can Be Made

1. People can turn into criminals anywhere in the Phunny Pharm, but the main place is in the jail, where the mean Heavy Metal Group plays and there is so much corruption.

Bad Guy Exit from the Phunny Pharm

1. Reformed criminal hero cleans up the Phunny Pharm by sweeping the criminals with her street sweeper.
2. Criminals can be kicked out of the country from jail and back into the ocean.

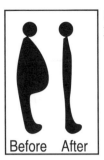

Diet

Diet is the first step of treatment because the decision to treat pharmacologically commits the patient to lifelong medication. The decision for treatment beyond diet needs to weigh the high cost, inconvenience, and side effects.

Bile Acid Binders

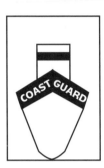

	Cholestyramine and Colestipol	**The Coast Guard**
N	Cholestyramine	The Coast Guard who stymies the criminals from coming ashore
	Colestipol	The cholesterol patrol
mech	Bind bile acids in the intestine and thereby prevent reabsorption	The Coast Guard prevents the criminals from coming ashore
	Because the liver makes bile acids from cholesterol, it increases removal of cholesterol from the blood.	Because new criminals are not coming into the country, there is more room in the jail, so the police department begins to round up more limos from the city.
	Lowers LDL cholesterol	Decreases the number of limos on the road
	Increases HDL	A bonus: more heroes to clean up the city
Tox	Bloating, constipation, and fat-soluble vitamin deficiencies ⇒ may be difficult to tolerate.	¢: from the mechanism of action
	May increase triglycerides	
Rt	PO only	Inherent in the mechanism of action
Uses	Hypercholesterolemia, except if patient has hypertriglyceridemia	
R_x/R_x	Impairs absorption of many drugs	Unfortunately, our two Coast Guard heroes can be indiscriminate and may prevent drugs and vitamins from entering the Phunny Pharm.
	May decrease vitamin K absorption → increase the anticoagulation effect of warfarin	

HMG-CoA Reductase Inhibitors   # Crime Preventors

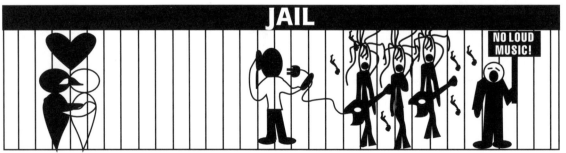

Lovastatin   Pravastatin   Simvastatin

N	All end in -vastatin:	They are all in the vast station preventing crime:
	Lovastatin	The lovers in the vast station
	Pravastatin	The preventor in the vast station
	Simvastatin	A sign man in the vast station
mech	Inhibit HMG-CoA reductase—the rate-limiting step of cholesterol biosynthesis → decreased synthesis of cholesterol in the liver and clearance of LDL from blood by the liver.	They prevent normal people from being reduced to criminals by this mean heavy metal group.
	→ ↓ LDL	Because of these crime preventors, the jail also takes limos off of the Phunny Pharm roads.
	→ ↓ total cholesterol	Decreases numbers of all criminals
Tox	Minimal; rare myositis and increased LFTs*	The jail may be damaged.
	Rare lupus-like syndrome	The heavy metal group has a wolf that may attack the crime preventors.
Uses	Hypercholesterolemia	Prevents the formation of criminals
R$_x$/R$_x$	Enhance anticoagualation of warfarin	
	Should not be used with the fibric acid derivatives → increased myositis	The crime preventors and gem fibber do not get along because gem fibber likes heavy metal (see Gemgibrozil below).

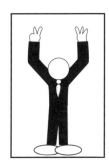

Nicotinic acid

Nixon

mech	Exact mechanism unclear, but does all of the right things in regard to the profile:	Nixon learned his lesson; now he does all of the right things.
	→ ↓ LDL, plasma triglycerides, and total cholesterol	Smashes limos, VWs (his fingers say "V-W"), and all criminals
	→ ↑ HDL	A bonus: more heroes to clean up the city
Tox	Flushing	Nixon blushes after he is presented with a street sweeper for cleaning up the city.
Uses	Hypercholesterolemia, hypertriglyceridemia, and mixed disorders	¢

Fibric Acids

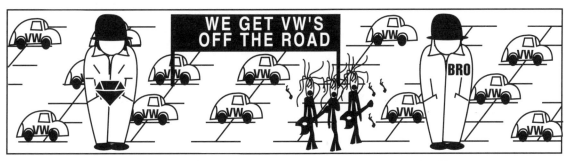

	Gemfibrozil	**Clofibrate**
N	Gemfibrozil	The gem fibber who steals VWs from the gangsters
	Clofibrate	Gem's brother—the collaborator fibber
mech	Decreases VLDL synthesis	Gem fibber and his collaborator steal VWs from the trios of gangsters.

*Liver function tests

	Increases <u>HDL</u>	They sell the VWs and buy street cleaners for the <u>heroes</u>.
Tox	May increase LDL	They may make a mistake and increase the number of limos on the road.
	Clofibrate may increase mortality from malignant and GI disease	
	Cholelithiasis*	
Uses	Clofibrate should only be used in severe hypertriglyceridemia after gemfibrozil	The collaborator should only be used if the gem fibber did not work.
R_x/R_x	Enhance anticoagualation of warfarin	
	Should not be used with HMG-CoA reductase inhibitor → increased myositis	The gem fibber likes heavy metal, so that he does not get along with the preventors of crime.

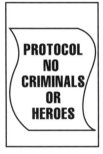

Probucol

mech   Decreases HDL and LDL

Uses   Hypercholesterolemia only, but rarely used

The Mayor's Strict <u>Protocol</u>

The protocol eliminates all criminals and heroes off of the street.

A protocol from a mayor seems to do no good anymore; therefore, it is not used in the Phunny Pharm.

---

*Cholelithiasis ⇒ gall stones.

Anticoagulation—Preventing or Removing Road Blocks

Robert Fulghum summarized coagulation better than any text in <u>It Was on Fire When I Lay Down on It</u>:

> "Blood equals emergency. But if you can somehow wire around your panic, an existential moment may come if you stand still and bleed a little into the sink. You will not die of this cut—you've cut your finger before . . .
>
> See, you won't bleed long. Your own interior Medic One takes care of the problem in an amazing way . . .
>
> You've stopped bleeding now. A sixteen-step protein cascade effect has built a dam and shut off the flow . . .
>
> If you'll just stand there patiently for five minutes these things will happen.
>
> Without your thinking or planning or organizing or trying.
>
> It's very beautiful, this blood of yours.
>
> It's very powerful and efficient.
>
> It's worthy of respect.
>
> It is life.
>
> Confirmed."*

This conveys the awesomeness of blood. The difficult task is to strip this cascade down to a minimum in order to understand the pharmacology of anticoagulation.

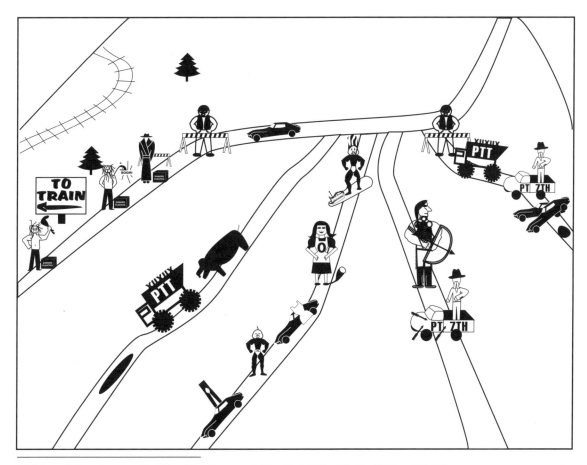

*Fulghum, Robert: <u>It was on Fire When I Lay Down on It.</u> New York, Villard Books, 1989, pp 117–119.

Picture Key

In this picture, the possibility of damage to the roads of the Phunny Pharm is introduced. Bleeding is represented by cars driving off damaged roads. In the body, control of bleeding is accomplished by platelets and the coagulation cascade, and in the Phunny Pharm, cars driving off the road are controlled by Corvettes and road blocks put up by the police and reinforced by the road block building crew.

Vessels	The Phunny Pharm Roads
Blood	Things that drive or are simply on the road
Clot	Road block to prevent cars from driving on the damaged road
Damaged vessels	Damage to the roads
Platelets	Corvettes driven by police
Coagulation factors	Cement that solidifies road blocks

Introduction to Coagulation

Definitions

Clot ⇒ solidification of blood to stop hemorrhage

Primary hemostasis ⇒ interaction of platelets with vessel walls following damage to prevent further blood loss. This results in the formation of a platelet plug.

Secondary hemostasis ⇒ activation of coagulation factors, and finally fibrin, to stabilize the platelet plug

Coagulation ⇒ the sequential activation of the blood coagulation factors, resulting in formation of an insoluble clot. This occurs by the activation of the intrinsic and extrinsic pathways, activation of the common pathway, formation of thrombin, and ultimately, of stable fibrin polymers.

Thrombus ⇒ a clot that includes platelets, fibrin, and additional blood cellular elements

Main Components of Clot Formation

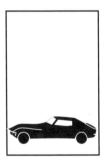

Platelets

Thromboxane A_2 is made by platelets → platelets to become "sticky."
They then stick together and form a temporary plug (i.e., platelet plug).

Remember that platelets lack a nucleus ⇒ their proteins cannot be replenished.

Corvettes Used as Road Blocks

Corvettes drive around on the roads and look for damage. If they see damage, they throw out a box of anchors → stick to other Corvettes (as sad as it may sound) and to the road. This creates a temporary road block to prevent cars from running off the road.

Corvettes have no spare tires and a limited number of boxes of anchors.

Coagulation Cascade

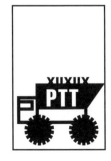

Intrinsic Pathway

Activated by abnormalities within the vessel wall

Activation of factors XII → XI → IX results finally in activation of the common pathway.

Monitor PTT for function of this pathway.

Block with heparin.

Things That Solidify Road Blocks

The Peterbilt Dump Truck

Cement is dumped when it finds damage to the road.

The highest numbered factors

"Peterbilt" has two T's. A Peterbilt is also larger than a pickup truck, just as "PTT" has more letters (see next page) than "PT."

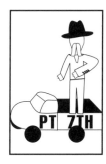

Extrinsic Pathway

Activated by abnormalities outside of the blood ⇒ by tissue factors

Factor <u>VII</u>, which requires vitamin <u>K</u> for its synthesis, activates factor X, and thereby activates the common pathway

Monitor <u>PT</u> for function of this pathway.

Block with <u>warfarin</u>.

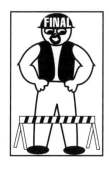

Common Pathway

Factor X is activated by extrinsic or intrinsic pathway → activation of thrombin → activation of <u>fibrin</u> → formation and stabilization of the platelet plug.

The Pickup Truck

Cement is dumped because of major damage to roads such as earthquakes or rock slides onto the road.

It only has to carry one <u>c</u>oagulation factor (<u>C</u>uster from the <u>7</u>th Calvary), so it is smaller.

"Pic<u>k</u>up" has a "K" in it, whereas "Peterbilt" does not.

Pickup <u>t</u>ruck has only one "T" in its name. A pickup truck is also smaller than a Peterbilt, just as "PT" has fewer letters than "PTT."

<u>Warfare</u> is after Custer.

Workers Making Road Blocks

There are many workers who build the road blocks from the ingredients in the trucks. When they are working, they ultimately order the <u>final</u> concrete worker (<u>fibrin</u>) to begin. He is responsible for maintaining solidification (with concrete) of the road blocks until repairs can be made to the road.

Main Components of Clot Prevention

<u>Endothelial integrity</u>:
    As long as vessels remain intact, <u>clots</u> will not form.

<u>Prostacyclin (PGI$_2$)</u>:
    Made by vascular endothelium via cyclooxygenase action on arachidonic acid. Endothelial cells have nuclei and can therefore replenish their proteins.
    Inhibit <u>platelet</u> stickiness
<u>Fibrinolysis</u>:
    Activation of <u>plasmin</u> → proteolysis of <u>fibrin</u> → dissolution of the <u>clot</u>

<u>Intact road</u>
As long as there is no damage, there is no need for <u>road blocks</u>.
<u>Prostaslick</u>
Prostaslick on the road
Unlimited amount of prostaslick for the roads

Prevents <u>Corvette</u> anchors from sticking
<u>To destroy the concrete road block</u>:
    <u>Plastic explosives</u> are used to blow up the <u>concrete road block</u>.

Thrombotic Problems

<u>Too little coagulation</u>:
    This causes excessive hemorrhage, with difficulties stopping bleeding.
<u>Too much coagulation</u>:
    Deep venous thrombosis (DVT)
    Pulmonary embolism
    Arterial emboli:
        Cerebrovascular accidents (CVA)
        Systemic emboli
    We can interfere with this system three ways:
        <u>Platelet</u> inhibitors
        Anticoagulants
        <u>Fibrinolytics</u>

This will not be discussed except as a side effect of the medications.
<u>Road blocks where they are not needed</u>:
    Can have road blocks in normal parking lots*
    Road blocks that are carried to the Airport†

Road blocks that cause damage to the University and the entire Phunny Pharm
Can prevent road blocks in three ways:
    Stop the <u>Corvettes</u>.
    Stop the trucks (Peterbilts or pickups).
    Break up the <u>concrete</u> in the road blocks.

---

*Rem: Veins are represented by the parking lots throughout the Phunny Pharm.
†Rem: The lungs are represented by the airport throughout the Phunny Pharm.

Platelets Inhibitors in General

N   Aspirin   The apron woman

            Sulfinpyrazone   The surfing pyromaniacs

            Dipyridamole   The diaper man

            Ticlopidine   Tie the clothespin.

mech   Decrease platelet aggregation.   Prevent the Corvettes from sticking.

Tox   Bleeding   They can inhibit the Corvettes too much.

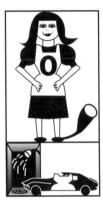

Aspirin

mech   Inhibit cyclooxygenase **irreversibly** → inhibition of TXA_2 synthesis, and therefore prevent activation of platelets

        Platelets cannot make more cyclooxygenase because they do not have nuclei.

        On the other hand, vessel endothelium have nuclei and can make more cyclooxygenase. This allows continued production of prostacyclin → inhibition of coagulation.

        Net effect is antiaggregatory.

Met   Kidney

        Follows zero-order kinetics

Tox   A "Barrier Breaker" ⇒ Also blocks cyclooxygenase in the stomach → inhibits production of prostaglandins which act as a barrier to acid → ulcers

        Causes asthma attacks in some patients with asthma.

Uses   Prevention of cerebrovascular accident, pulmonary embolism in patients who can't tolerate warfarin

        Prevention of myocardial infarction and even colon cancer

Apron Woman

Apron woman wraps her apron around Corvettes and permanently keeps them from throwing out their boxes of anchors.

The Corvettes cannot remove the aprons.

On the other hand, if the apron woman lays her aprons on the road to cover the prostaslick, they will not remain for long, and the prostaslick will be reexposed.

Net effect is to inhibit the Corvettes permanently and the roads temporarily, allowing the roads to be slippery.

She goes to shower when she is done.

She has a zero on her chest.

She also causes damage to the beach (GI mucosa; see p. 184).*

The apron woman is stepping on an airport tube.

The apron woman prevents damage to the Phunny Pharm University, airport, and train.

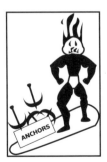

Sulfinpyrazone

mech   Reversibly inhibits cyclooxygenase (see explanation with aspirin)

A Surfing Pyromaniac

Borrows the boxes of anchors from the Corvettes to use when he surfs. When he is through with them, he returns them to the Corvettes (i.e., it is reversible).

---

*Please see page 192 for more information on ulcers.

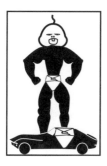

Dipyridamole

mech   Increases cAMP → decreased release of ADP from platelets → inhibition of platelet aggregation.

Uses   In patients with prosthetic valves in combination with other anticoagulation medications ⇒ not used alone

Diaper Man

Diaper man puts a diaper around Corvettes that keeps them from sticking together.

Diaper man is too young to attack the Corvettes alone.

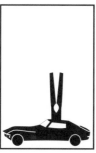

Ticlopidine

mech   Inhibits binding of fibrinogen to platelets

Tox   Nausea, diarrhea
      Severe neutropenia (1%)

Rt   PO

Uses   Prevention of CVA when patients have failed aspirin therapy or can't tolerate aspirin

Tie the Clothespin

Ties and pins the Corvettes

Only used to save the University* after the apron lady has failed or can't be used

Anticoagulants in General

N   Heparin
      Warfarin

mech   Decrease number or function of coagulation factors.

Uses   Prophylaxis against DVTs[†] and pulmonary emboli
      Heparin therapy requires monitoring of PTT.
      Warfarin therapy requires monitoring of PT.

The hippo that ruins Peterbilts
Warfare at Little Big Horn which destroys the 7th Calvary

Wreck the trucks and thereby prevent road blocks from being formed.

Prevent road blocks in parking lots and the Phunny Pharm airport.
The hippo ruins the Peterbilt truck.
The warfare wrecks the pickup truck.

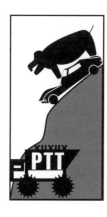

Heparin

mech   Mainly inhibits intrinsic pathway.
      Large negative charge allows it to bind and activate antithrombin III → inhibition of thrombin. Therefore, it is a potent indirect inhibitor of thrombin.
      Also inactivates IX, X, XI, and XII

Dist   Does not cross placenta or into maternal milk

Met   Liver and uptake by macrophages and endothelial cells

Tox   **Bleeding**
      Monitor PTT
      Thrombocytopenia
      Allergy
      Protamine sulfate can be used as an antidote, as it complexes with heparin, inactivating it.

Hippo that Ruins the Peterbilt

The hippo ruins Peterbilts.

Waits at the damaged roads, and ruins the Peterbilt, so that it cannot dump its cement (XII,XI,IX,X)

The hippo stays away from babies.

The Phunny Pharm police take the hippo off of the roads.

May ruin too many Peterbilts
Ruins the Peterbilt, so monitor PTT
The hippo can also ruin Corvettes.

A pro team safari can be used to get rid of the hippos.

---

*Rem: The CNS is represented by the University throughout the Phunny Pharm.
[†]DVT ⇒ deep venous thrombosis.

Rt	IV and Q only	
Uses	Mainly used for initiation of anticoagulation therapy	Hippos only stick around until the warfare breaks out; then they leave.
	Used in pregnancy	These hippos do not bother babies.

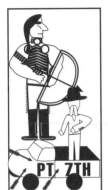

Warfarin

Warfare at Little Big Horn

mech	Mainly inhibits the <u>extrinsic</u> pathway	The <u>pickup</u> is the only truck that is worried about the warfare, because it is the only one that is small enough to be damaged.
	Inhibits activation of vitamin K dependent factors, thereby preventing the <u>liver</u> from manufacturing active clotting factors by depletion of vitamin K $\Rightarrow$ prothrombin, II, VII, IX, X	When the pickup truck hears there is warfare at the Little Big Horn, it refuses to leave the Phunny Pharm <u>police station</u>.
	Factor VII has the shortest $t_{1/2}$; therefore, it is depleted first.	2, 7, 9, and 10* synthesis are inhibited. 7th Calvary in the back of the pickup are glad to stay in the police station.
Met	Hepatic by the P-450 system	
$t_{1/2}$	Highly variable	
Tox	**Bleeding**	The warfare may destroy too many pickups.
	Inhibits bone mineralization in babies; therefore, not allowed in pregnancy	Babies should not be exposed to warfare.
	PT must be monitored.	Pickup truck has only one "T" in it.
	Vitamin K is the antidote.	
Rt	PO	
R_x/R_x	Many	

Fibrinolytics in General

N	End in -kinase	
	Urokinase	The <u>urinator</u>
	Streptokinase	The <u>stripper</u>
	<u>Tissue</u> <u>plasminogen</u> <u>activator</u> (TPA)	<u>The</u> <u>preferred</u> <u>agent</u>
mech	Dissolve <u>clots</u> by digestion of <u>fibrin</u>.	Blow up <u>concrete</u> <u>road blocks</u>
	Converts plasminogen to <u>plasmin</u>, which proteolyzes fibrin	Use <u>plastic</u> explosives to destroy road blocks
Tox	If ischemic area is necrotic, then fibrinolytics can cause hemorrhage into necrotic area as clot is dissolved.	
Rt	IV	
Uses	Treatment of myocardial infarction by dissolution of thrombi in coronary vasculature causing the ischemia	Specialize in road blocks at the Phunny Pharm train and . . .
	Treatment of massive pulmonary embolism	. . . at the road to the airport.

---

*To remember these, picture them in the back of the truck, remember 2 + 7 = 9, 10, or just repeat it a few times (i.e., "2, 7, 9, 10").

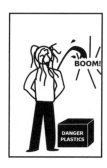

Urokinase

mech   Complexes and activates plasminogen
        systemically

Uses   Can use in people with antibodies to
        or allergy to streptokinase
        Intracoronary in the cardiac catheter
        laboratory
        Not used systemically

Urinator Who Urinates Plastics

Doesn't care where he urinates, but
    wherever he does the plastics in his
    urine explode concrete
If the stripper cannot be tolerated,
    then the urinator may be.
Urinator is used mainly on the roads
    leading to the Phunny Pharm train.
Don't want a urinator running all over
    the place

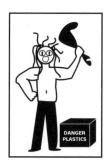

Streptokinase

mech   Activates plasminogen → plasmin by
        direct proteolysis systemically

$t_{1/2}$ Has a long lytic state compared to
        tissue plasminogen activator

Tox   Antigenic

The Stripper Who Uses Plastics

The stripper doesn't care where in the
    body he plants his plastics.

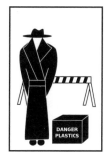

Tissue Plasminogen Activator (TPA)

N   TPA

mech   Preferentially acts upon fibrin-bound
        plasminogen ⇒ plasminogen at
        the clot

Met   Liver

Tox   Expensive

Uses   Myocardial infarction
        Heparin must be used after TPA
        because of short lytic period

The Preferred Agent

The preferred agent sneaks up to the
    road blocks and plants his
    explosives.
He is a professional ⇒ only plants his
    plastics at sites of road blocks.

The police* send him to the jail.

---

*Rem: The liver is represented by the jail and police station throughout the Phunny Pharm.

Inflammatory Mediators—Introduction

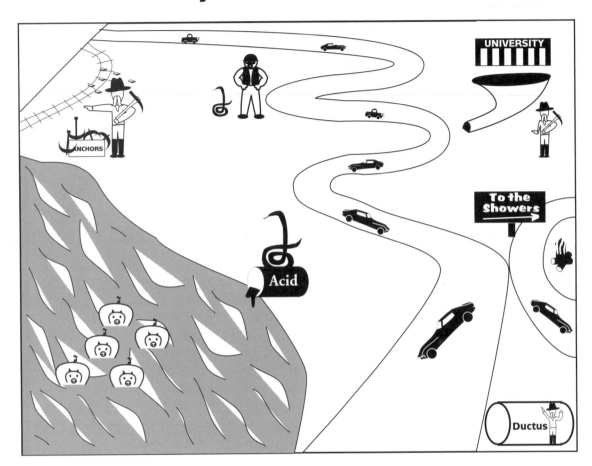

Picture Key

Cyclooxygenase	Cyclooxygenase man
Prostaglandins	Prospector who protects the land
Thromboxanes	Throw out a box of anchors
Histamine	The hissing snake
Platelets	Corvettes
Vasculature	The Phunny Pharm roads
Bronchi	Tubes leading to the airport
Gastrointestinal tract	The ocean
GI mucosa	The beach
Hydrogen ions ⇒ acid	Hogs
Bicarbonate	Bees
CNS	The Phunny Pharm University
Pain	Weather causing damage somewhere in the Phunny Pharm
Inflammation	Fire in the Phunny Pharm

Eicosanoids

Eicosanoids are metabolites derived from the polyunsaturated fatty acid, arachidonic acid. Arachidonic acid is esterified in membrane phospholipids. After it is liberated by phospholipase A_2, it is quickly converted to eicosanoids specific to the tissue in which the arachidonic acid is freed. This specificity is due to the enzymes located in the tissue.

Cyclooxygenase converts arachidonic acid to prostaglandin H_2 (PGH_2).

PGH_2 is then converted to other prostaglandins, PGD_2, PGE_2, PGF_2, or prostacyclin (PGI_2).

PGH_2 can be converted to thromboxanes (TXA_2, or TXB_2).

Lipoxygenase converts arachidonic acid to the leukotrienes.

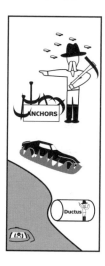

	Prostaglandins in General	**Prospector Protecting the Land**
mech	Have actions throughout the body:	
	CV ⇒ some → vasodilation, some → vasoconstriction	
	Blood ⇒ prostacyclin antiaggregatory produced by endothelial walls.	Prostaslick that is placed on the roads prevents Corvettes from sticking to the roads.
	Thromboxane A_2 → pro-aggregatory, produced by platelets	Cyclooxygenase man can throw a box of anchors out of the Corvette → Corvette to stick to the road.
	Lungs ⇒ bronchial dilation	Prospector keeps airport tubes open.
	GI ⇒ stomach ⇒ ↑ barrier to acid and ↓ acid secretion	Prospector protects the land at the beach by building a barrier that prevents the pigs from hurting it and by preventing the hogs from going into the ocean.
	Intestines ⇒ ↑ secretion (e.g., HCO_3^-) to neutralize acid; can → diarrhea	In some parts of the ocean, the prospector sends bees out to drown the pigs.
	Inflammation ⇒ ↑ pain and edema	Prospector can drop the anchors → pain.
Met	Thought to occur in the tissue of origin, but IV administration of a prostaglandin shows extensive metabolism in liver and lung	
$t_{1/2}$	Seconds	¢: Because of extensive metabolism
Rt	Not usually parenteral because nonspecificity of actions and rapid metabolism	
Uses	Maintain patent ductus arteriosus	The prospector makes his way to the ductus and holds it open.*
	Induce labor	
	Constriction of uterus	
	Form a barrier to acid in stomach ⇒ prevent ulcers, especially ulcers of NSAIDs	Protects the beach with his bees and pigs especially from the ships

---

*Adapted from an analogy used by Frank Fitzpatrick, Ph.D.

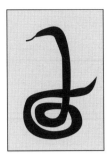

Histamine in General

mech   Stored in mast cells in skin, mucous
       membranes, GI mucosa, lungs, and
       basophils

       Released in hypersensitivity reactions
       or for stimulation of acid secretion
       in the GI

       Histamine binds H_1 or H_2 receptor:
       CV (H_1 receptors) $\Rightarrow$ largest effect
       is upon the vasculature;
       $\rightarrow$ vasodilation, $\uparrow$ vascular
       permeability, $\downarrow$ BP
       Nerve endings (H_1 receptors) $\Rightarrow$
       itching and <u>pain</u>
       GI (H_2 receptors) $\Rightarrow$ secretion of
       <u>acid</u>, pepsin, and intrinsic factor

Uses   Histamine is not used, but histamine
       receptor antagonists have
       widespread use.

Hissing Snake

The snake is all over the body.

Causes the dumping of acid into the
ocean

Places where the snake can act:

Hissing snake can scare the road
workers into building more roads.

Hissing snake can make it <u>hail</u>* <u>on
the University</u>.

Can chase the <u>pigs</u> into the ocean

Only try to get rid of the snake

---

*Rem: Pain is represented by weather throughout the Phunny Pharm.

Nonsteroidal Antiinflammatory Drugs—Boats at the Beach

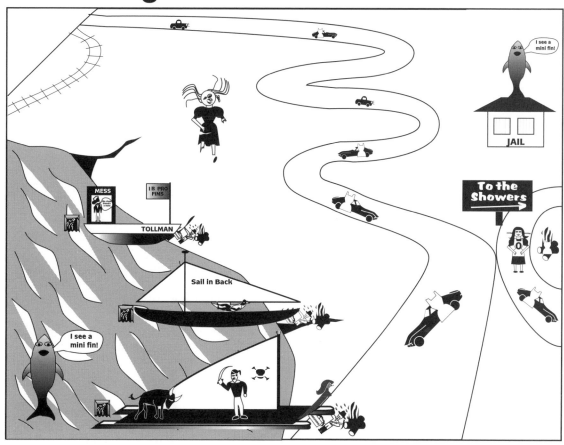

Nonsteroidal Antiinflammatory Drugs in General

N	Aspirin	Apron woman
	Other NSAIDs	Three ships
mech	Weak acids	
	Inhibit cyclooxygenase → inhibition of prostaglandin synthesis	Stop the prospector.
Dist	Highly protein bound	
$t_{1/2}$	Main difference between drugs lie in the pharmacokinetics	Their size in the pictures ⇒ the larger the boat, the longer the half-life
Tox	Gastric irritation and bleeding ⇒ "**barrier breakers**" ⇒ they destroy the barrier that protects the intestinal lining from the acid	They cause damage at the beach.
Rt	PO except ketorolac	They get into the Phunny Pharm via the ocean.
Uses	All can be used as antiinflammatory, analgesic, and/or antipyretic, although the doses required for antiinflammatory effects are higher.	All fight fires prevent hail from damaging the University, and turn off the oven.

R_x/R_x Protein displacement of other highly protein
              bound drugs—e.g., antithrombotics
              Compete for reabsorption with organic anions
              in the kidney

Aspirin   ## Apron Woman

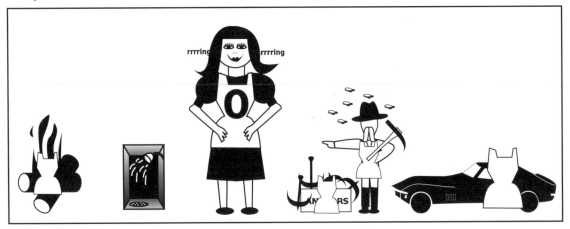

mech	Acetylates and thereby **irreversibly** inhibits cyclooxygenase → inhibits prostaglandin and thromboxane synthesis	Apron woman wraps her apron around the cyclooxygenase man and prevents him from throwing his boxes of anchors.

mech   Acetylates and thereby **irreversibly** inhibits
       cyclooxygenase → inhibits prostaglandin
       and thromboxane synthesis

Blood:

   Platelets ⇒ inhibit thromboxane synthesis
   → prevents activation of platelets.
   Because aspirin is irreversible and
   platelets do not have nuclei, they can
   not make more cyclooxygenase →
   permanent inactivation of the platelet.

   Vessel endothelium ⇒ there is a nucleus
   and can therefore make more
   cyclooxygenase. This allows continued
   production of prostacyclin → inhibition
   of coagulation.

   Net effect is antiaggregatory.

Apron woman wraps her apron around the
cyclooxygenase man and prevents him from
throwing his boxes of anchors.

On the Phunny Pharm roads:

   The Corvettes cannot remove the aprons →
   keep them from throwing the boxes of
   anchors → permanently prevents them
   from sticking to the road.

   The apron woman lays her aprons on the road
   to cover the prostaslick; they will not
   remain for long, and the prostaslick will be
   reexposed → the Corvettes do not stick to
   the road.

   Net effect is to inhibit the Corvettes
   permanently and the roads **temporarily**

   Antipyretic
   Analgesia

Met   Follows zero-order kinetics
   Renal

Tox   GI—epigastric pain, ulceration
   Hypersensitivity—rash, bronchospasm;
   therefore, should be avoided in some
   asthmatics (up to 10% of asthmatics have
   this hypersensitivity).
   Blood—↑ bleeding time

   Renal—low doses ⇒ competes with uric acid
   secretion → ↑ serum uric acid
   Extremely high doses ⇒ competes with uric
   acid reabsorption →↓ serum uric acid
   Reye syndrome in children and adolescents
   in the presence of viral infection and fever;
   results in 35% mortality

Apron woman puts out the fire.
She prevents hail from hitting the University.
Apron woman has a zero on her chest.
She takes a shower when she is done.
Apron woman damages the beach.

By blocking the Corvettes → cars to run off
   the roads

Apron woman is mean, she may feed spoiled rye
   bread to children.

Salicylism—tinnitus and vertigo

Acute overdose → hyperventilation → respiratory alkalosis; then becomes metabolic acidosis

Treated by alkalinizing urine → ↑ secretion into urine

Uses   **Many** uses: antipyretic, analgesia, prevention of stroke, myocardial infarction, anticoagulation when warfarin cannot be used, prevention of colon cancer . . .

Her ears are ringing and she is dizzy.

¢: Since aspirin is a weak acid. Please practice going through the physiology.

Other Nonsteroidal Antiinflammatories in General

N   Short acting:

    Tolmetin

    Ibuprofen

    Indomethacin

    Meclofenamate

  Intermediate acting:

    Naproxen

    Sulindac

  Long acting:

    Piroxicam

    Phenylbutazone

mech   **Reversibly** inhibit cyclooxygenase

Tox   Same side effects as for aspirin, but usually less severe

    GI ulcers

    Renal failure

The smallest ship:

    Ship's name is "Tollman."

    "I be pro fins" hangs from a banner.

    The captain likes to eat in the mess.

    Captain says "me close friend's a mate."

Medium-sized ship—a sailboat:

    The napping oxen sleep on the deck of this ship.

    The sail is in the back of the ship.

Biggest ship—a huge catamaran:

    The pirate's catamaran

    The catamaran has a funny beauty of its own.

Temporarily stop cyclooxygenase man

They maneuver their ships on the roads to do the same things as apron woman, but only temporarily.

They damage the beach as they go ashore

They damage the showers.

Short-Acting NSAIDs   The Smallest Ship

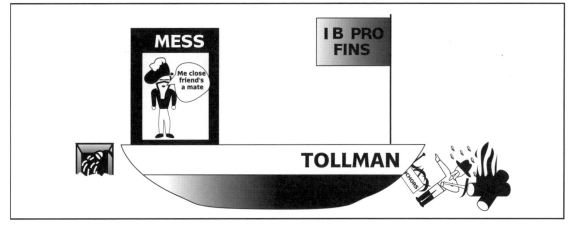

N   Tolmetin

    Ibuprofen

    Indomethacin

    Meclofenamate

Tox   Indomethacin ⇒ more commonly causes ulcers and more likely to be nephrotoxic

Ship's name is "Tollman."

"I be pro fins" hangs from a banner.

The captain likes to eat in the mess.

Captain says "me close friend's a mate."

Intermediate-Acting NSAIDs

Medium-Sized Ship—a Sailboat

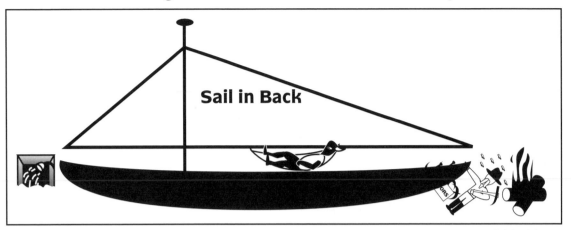

N   <u>Naproxen</u>
        <u>Sulindac</u>

The <u>napping oxen</u> sleep on the deck of this ship.
The <u>sail</u> is <u>in the back</u> of the ship.

Long-Acting NSAIDs

Biggest Ship— a Huge Catamaran

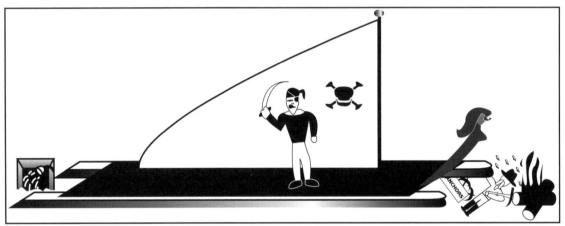

mech	<u>Piroxicam</u>
	<u>Phenylbutazone</u>
	<u>Ketorolac</u>
Rt	Ketorolac is the only <u>parenteral</u> NSAID.
Tox	Phenylbutazone ⇒ agranulocytosis and rare irreversible aplastic anemia
Uses	Ketorolac is a very effective analgesic; is at least equivalent to an acetaminophen/ codeine combination

The <u>pirate's catamaran</u>
Catamaran has a <u>funny beauty of its own</u>.
A <u>key</u> <u>toro</u> in <u>back</u>
The toro is very <u>muscular</u>.

Other Analgesics

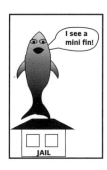

Acetaminophen

mech	Analgesic
	Antipyretic
	Mechanism unknown, but it does not inhibit cyclooxygenase ⇒ it is **not** an antiinflammatory agent
Met	Hepatic conjugation
Tox	Hepatic toxicity in overdose—treated with N-acetylcysteine ⇒ provides sulfhydryl groups
Rt	PO or per rectum
Uses	Antipyresis
	Analgesia

"I See a Mini Fin"

Prevents damage from bad storms with his body

Can turn off the oven

The fish does not touch the cyclooxygenase man.

He is sitting on the jail in the picture.

If there are too many of these fish in the Phunny Pharm, their weight will crush the jail.

The fish comes from the ocean.

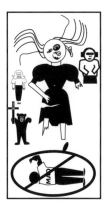

Tramadol

mech	Binds to μ-opioid receptors → analgesia
	Inhibits reuptake of norepinephrine and serotonin
Tox	Nausea, dizziness, constipation, sedation, and headache
	Expensive
Rt	PO
Uses	Analgesia
	Little potential for addiction
R_x/R_x	Should not be used in patients taking monoamine oxidase inhibitors.

Trauma Doll

She works on the weather station workers.

She keeps the Norepi cross and Sarah around.

She does not get along with the MAO bouncer.

Antiulcers—Beach Damage Prevention

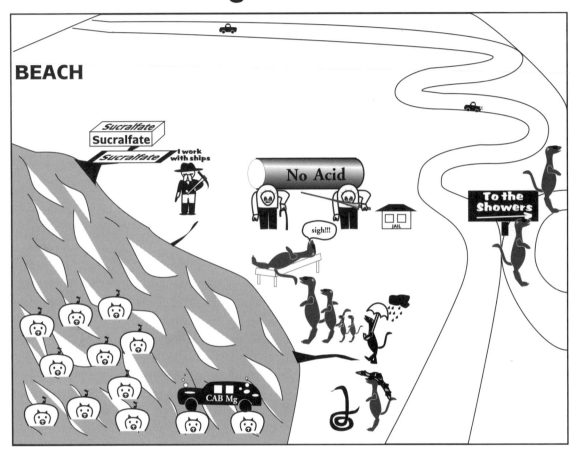

Picture Key

The beach represents the mucosal wall of the gastrointestinal tract. This beach appears in many other pictures as an entrance into the Phunny Pharm, but here damage is occuring from acid. This acid is represented by the hogs on the beach who are sent out into the ocean by the "acid tube" seen in other pictures. Things that stop this tube decrease the acid produced, and things that drown hogs are things that decrease acid in the GI tract.

Gastrointestinal tract	Ocean
Mucosal wall of the GI tract	The beach
$\underline{H}^+$	$\underline{H}$ogs
$\underline{K}^+$	$\underline{P}$igs
HCO_3^- (bicarbonate)	$\underline{B}$ees that drown the hogs $\Rightarrow$ neutralize acid
Parietal cell	The <<acid tube>> that is dumping the hogs and the pigs into the ocean
Stimulation of the parietal cell	Something camps on top of the tube.
$\underline{P}$rostaglandin	The old $\underline{p}$rospector on the beach who protects it
The normal barrier to acid	A barrier fortified by the prospector that prevents damage to the beach
Ulcer	Damage to the beach

Histamine
Antiulcer medications

Hissing snake
Things that stop beach destruction or decrease the number of hogs sent out into the ocean

Acid Secretion in the Parietal Cell of the Gastric Mucosa

Proton pump in the gastric parietal cells $\Rightarrow$ H^+/K^+ ATPase pumps H^+ into the stomach.
Stimulated by $\uparrow$ in cAMP within the parietal cell:

Hogs/pigs are sent out into the ocean by the acid tube on the beach.
Things camping on top of the acid tube increase acid:

H_2-receptor stimulation by histamine

Hissing snakes will camp on top of the acid tube

Muscarinic receptor activation by Ach

The 3 musketeer cubs camp on top of the acid tube

Gastrin receptor stimulation by gastrin
Inhibited by $\downarrow$ in cAMP within the parietal cell:

Things that chase the animals off of the acid tube $\rightarrow$ decreased acid from the tube:

Prostaglandin (PGE_2)

The prospector decreases the hogs sent into the ocean.

H_2-Receptor Antagonists: The Mongooses

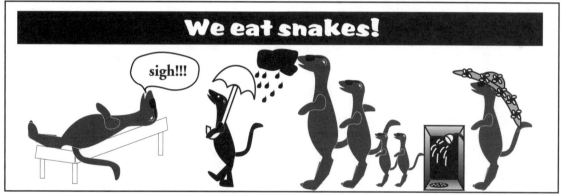

		Cimetidine	Ranitidine	Famotidine	Nizatidine

N | All end in -tidine

Cimetidine
Ranitidine
Famotidine
Nizatidine

Two mongoose who love to dine on hissing snakes:
The mongoose on the beach who sighs
The mongoose upon whom it always rains
A family of mongooses at the beach
A mongoose wearing a nice hat on the beach

mech | Blocks acid secretion due to any cause:

Competitively inhibit H_2-receptors $\rightarrow$ prevention of stimulation of acid secretion $\rightarrow$ $\downarrow$ **acid production** in the stomach by parietal cells in both fasting and nonfasting states
Little or no effect on H_1-receptors

Each mongoose loves to stop the acid tube, no matter the cause:
They jump onto the tube and prevent snakes from camping on the tube $\rightarrow$ decreased acid secretion into the ocean.

The mongooses remain at the beach where there are H_2 snakes. They never eat H_1 snakes in the nose.*

Met | Unchanged in urine

The mongoose go to the showers when they are through at the beach.

Tox | Minimal
Leukopenia and neutropenia
CNS $\Rightarrow$ headache, dizziness

¢: They are selective for H_2-receptors.

*See page 196.

Rt	PO or IV	¢: From the mechanism and site of action
Uses	Duodenal and gastric ulcers	They will stop production of acid no matter what the cause is.
	Second-line agents for Zollinger-Ellison syndrome (gastrinoma) after proton-pump inhibitors	
	Reflux esophagitis	
R_x/R_x	**Cimetidine inhibits cytochrome P-450** system ⇒ slows metabolism of warfarin, phenytoin, theophylline, phenobarbital, many benzos, propranolol, nifedipine, digitoxin, quinidine, mexiletine, and tricyclic antidepressants	Very important to remember.

Direct Inhibition of H⁺ Pump   ## The Old Men

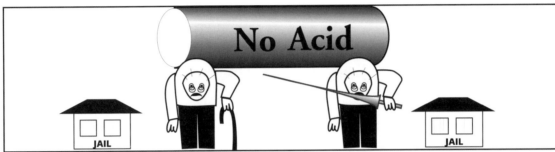

Omeprazole   **Lansoprazole**

N	Omeprazole	Ol' Mep who raises the hole
	Lansoprazole	The old man with a lance who raises the hole
mech	Inhibits acid production by the H^+/K^+ ATPase in the parietal cell by binding directly to the enzyme.	Ol' Mep and the man with the lance raise the hole so the tube cannot send hogs out into the ocean; therefore, acid production is stopped.
	It has little effect on total volume and other gastric secretions, or gastric motility.	
	Reduces the production of acid by the stomach by 85–95%	Ol' Mep is incredible at stopping the acid production.
Met	Hepatic	They both are sent to jail after they are through.
Tox	GI ⇒ nausea, emesis, diarrhea	
	Causes gastric carcinoid tumors in rats —not found in humans	
Uses	Same uses as for H_2-receptor antagonists but **more** effective	Ol' Mep and the old man with the lance are so good, they will work on any cause of acid production.
	Zollinger-Ellison syndrome	

Others

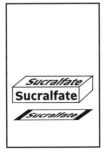

Sucralfate   **Sucralfate Gum**

mech	Acid within the stomach → polymerization and crosslinking between sucralfate molecules → sticks to ulcers	Hogs in the ocean take the gum, chew it, and use it to cover the damaged area of the beach.
	Less importantly, stimulates production of prostaglandin ↑ barrier to acid	The prospector loves gum, so he tries to get more gum.
Tox	Constipation and dry mouth	Gums up bowel movements
Rt	PO	¢: Site of action

Uses   May work better for duodenal ulcers than for gastric ulcers

R_x/R_x Antacids can prevent effectiveness of sucralfate by inhibiting acid activation.

¢: Acid is needed in order to activate sucralfate.

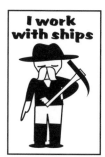

Misoprostol

mech   Analog of $PGE_1 \rightarrow$ inhibit acid secretion and $\uparrow$ mucus and HCO_3^- producton

Tox   Abdominal cramping, diarrhea

Rt   PO

Uses   Prevent ulcer formation in patients taking aspirin or other NSAIDS

The <u>Ol'</u> <u>Miser</u> <u>Prospector</u>

The old miser prospector is a good friend of the main prospector who protects the beach, so he does the same thing that the prospector does: stops hogs from going into the ocean and makes his bees go out to drown the pigs already there.

¢: Site of action

Prevent damage to the beach by the ships

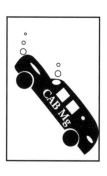

Antacids in General

N   First letters spell CAB Mg: <u>C</u>aCO_3, <u>A</u>l(OH)$_3$, Na<u>H</u>CO_3, (<u>B</u>icarb) <u>M</u>g(OH)$_2$

mech   Bases that directly neutralize gastric acid

Tox   All can $\rightarrow$ a metabolic alkalosis
<u>C</u>aCO_3 and Al(OH)$_3$ $\rightarrow$ <u>c</u>onstipation
Mg(OH)$_2$ $\rightarrow$ diarrhea
NaHCO_3 $\rightarrow$ $\uparrow$ Na load

Rt   PO

Uses   Peptic ulcers

R_x/R_x May change bioavailability of PO drugs and change the rate of excretion of drugs in the urine

The <u>CAB</u> of <u>Mg</u>

A floating CAB made of magnesium that floats in the ocean and drowns hogs

The CAB Mg drowns the hogs directly.

¢

¢: By site of action

They prevent damage to the beach.

¢: Because they will change the pH at both sites and therefore change absorption and excretion

Antihistamines—Things That Eat Snakes in the Nose

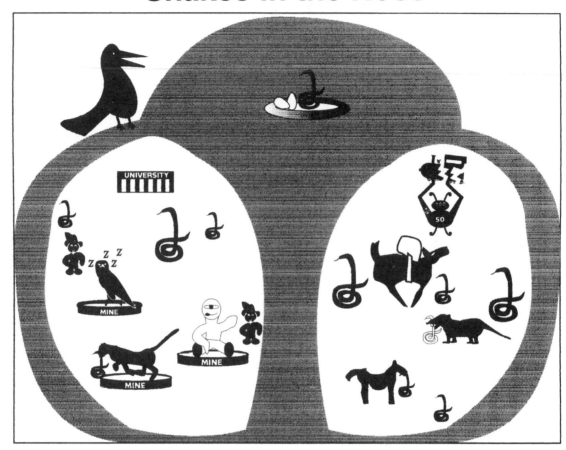

Antihistamines in General

In this picture, we are no longer at the beach, but we go to another area of the Phunny Pharm in which the histamine hissing snakes live. This place is your favorite and mine—the nose. In the nose, histamine wreaks havoc with our allergies and can make us miserable. Therefore, the antihistamines are things that eat or dispose of the hissing snake.

N   Traditional antihistamines

         Nonsedating antihistamines

mech   Competitively inhibit H_1 receptors

         Blocks H_1 receptor effects, which include edema, itching, capillary permeability, motion sickness

Met   Hepatic

Rt   PO/IV

The things that eat snakes and cause drowsiness all have mines in their pictures, and they can be seen in a different side of the nose from the nonsedating antihistamines in the big picture.

Things that eat or kill the hissing snake in the nose.

Keep hissing snakes from biting the roads and making them leak.

All may be put in jail.

Uses   **Symptomatic** treatment of allergies ⇒ relief from rhinitis, itching, and rashes

Decrease motion sickness

Vertigo

These things only kill the snakes once they are in the nose, but they do not prevent the snakes from arriving.

They also prevent the snakes from getting to your mind and making you dizzy.

Traditional Antihistamines in General (A Few of the Many)

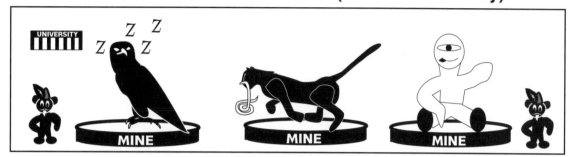

Diphenhydramine   **Pyrilamine**   **Chlorpheniramine**

N   They all end in -amine

       Diphenhydramine
       Pyrilamine
       Chlorpheniramine

Dist   Tertiary amines cross BBB very easily.

Tox   Cause sedation and depression due to activation of H_1 receptor blockade in the brain
       Chlorpheniramine has the least sedation.

Also have antimuscarinic effects ⇒ may decrease secretions, cause urinary retention
       Pyrilamine has the least antimuscarinic side effects.

Uses   Diphenhydramine also used for sedation

When the snakes slither across the mines, they blow up.

A dumb falcon who cannot fly hides the mines.
A really mean panther lays mines
A funny cyclops named Chlor lays mines
All of these animals have mortarboards.
These animals fall asleep while they wait for their mines to blow up a snake.

The cyclops has only one eye, so he must keep it open to watch for the snakes ⇒ no napping.
They may blow up the three musketeer cubs with their mines.
The really mean panther likes to eat snakes only. Eating cubs is too easy.
The dumb falcon will also put you to sleep.

Nonsedating Antihistamines in General

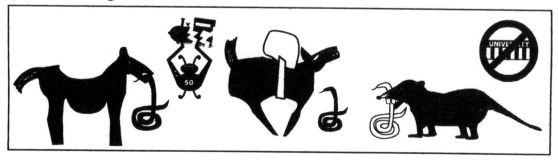

Terfenadine   **Astemizole**   **Loratadine**

N   Terfenadine
       Astemizole
       Loratadine

A tuff old nag* who likes to dine on snakes
The ass that is timid but can still kill snakes
A lowly rat loves to dine on snakes.

---

*Nag ⇒ an old horse.

mech	Little or no sedation	They are all wide awake.
Dist	All are quaternary amines ⇒ do not cross BBB	They are all timid and will not go to the University.
Tox	No antimuscarinic or sedative effects.	Don't affect the 3 musketeer cubs.
	Terfenadine and astemizole may cause arrhythmias when used in combination with <u>eythromycin</u> or cisapride.	<u>Free throw mycin</u> is holding a broken train.
	More expensive	¢: These are newer and have less side effects.
R_x/R_x	Arrhythmias—especially **torsades de pointes,** when used with <u>erythromycin</u> and others.	They may run the train off the tracks if they get together with <u>Free-Throw Mycin.</u>

Antihistamine That Works by Prophylaxis

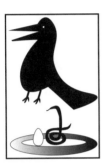

Cromolyn

The <u>Crow</u> Who Eats Snake Eggs

mech	Inhibits mediator release from mast cells	The crow prevents the snakes from leaving their nest.
	Decreases hyperreactivity of the airway	Prevents the airport tubes from closing
	No bronchodilating effects	The crow does nothing to the airport tubes themselves.
Tox	Minimal—generally benign	Crow is nice.
Rt	Aerosol	The crow can fly.
Uses	**Prophylaxis**—especially in allergic asthma	Prevents the snakes from leaving their nests

Asthma—Keeping Airport Tubes Open

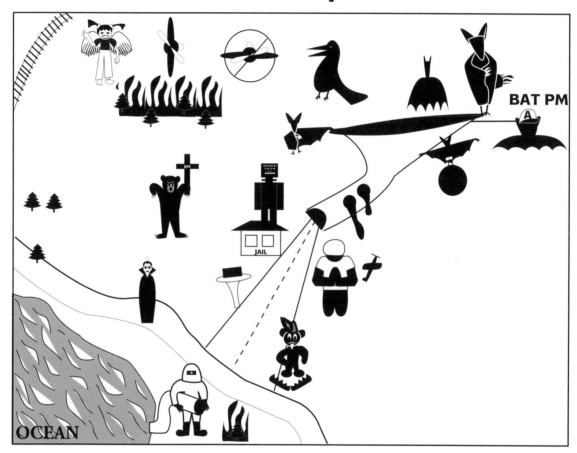

Asthma is an intermittent and reversible disease that is manifested by airway obstruction. An inflammatory reaction causes changes in the airway that decrease the flow of air into the lungs. These changes include inflammatory cell infiltration, epithelial disruption, and an exaggerated bronchoconstrictor response to many insults. These may include anything from specific triggers, such as allergens, to something as nonspecific as cold air. While the pathophysiology of this disease is complex and not fully understood, many targets for therapy exist.

Therapy Targets

Avoid the trigger

Prophylactic: Block the inflammation that contributes to airway hyperresponsivity.
Symptomatic: Treat the hyperresponsiveness of the airway.

Unless avoidance interferes with life, as when the trigger is exercise, or interferes with sleep
Used in people with recurrent asthma or asthma that interferes with activities or sleep
Used in people free of disease for long periods of time and for acute dyspnea in more serious disease

Picture Key (Pathogenesis of Asthma)

Bronchoconstriction	Decreased air space in tunnels for planes to enter
Inflammation in the airway	Fire in the air space
Inflammatory mediator release	Pyromaniacs (i.e., fire starters) in the lung tubes
Epithelial damage	Burnt walls of tunnel
Increased vascular permeability	Raining into the tunnels

β-Agonists in General (see also sympathomimetic chapter)

N	β-agonists	Things that scare bats, or bats and vampires.
mech	Stimulation of β_2-receptors $\rightarrow$ smooth muscle relaxation	Scare the bats, and they do things to the tunnels that $\rightarrow$ them to remain open.
	Decrease vascular permeability	They help to keep the rain out of the tunnel.
$t_{1/2}$	Most are short	Bats fly very fast.
Tox	Toxicities are mostly due to activation of β_1-receptors. Even the most β_2-selective are not exclusive of β_1-receptor activity.	Even though they scare mainly bats, they all can scare vampires when they get into the bloodstream.
	Tachycardia	The vampires after they are scared make the heart train run faster in fear.
	Tremor	Vampires on the streets, after they are scared, make everybody tremor with fear.
Rt	Aerosol	All of these things can fly and therefore enter through the airport.
	Most can be used PO or parenterally, but usually tolerated less well with questionable increased benefit over aerosol	
Uses	Most potent and most rapidly acting bronchodilators, so they can be used for acute bronchospasm	They can fly faster than other things opening the tubes to the airport.

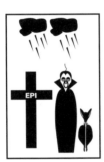

Catecholamines | Scaring Vampires and Bats

N	Epinephrine	The cross with epi written on it
	Isoproterenol	An ice storm that scares vampires and bats
mech	Epinephrine is α- and β-agonist.	The cross scares antelope, vampires, and bats.
	Isoproterenol is β nonselective	The ice storm scares vampires and bats only.
Dist	Mainly remain in lungs when delivered by aerosol but systemic absorption and nonselectivity allow for side effects	They scare bats when they fly into the airways, but if they get into the blood then they begin to scare vampires and cause side effects.
Tox	Mostly due to β_1-crossover Cardiac stimulation	If they get into the blood, then they will become vampires and will scare the Phunny Pharm train* to work harder.
Rt	Aerosol IV/SQ.	They can fly.
Uses	Epinephrine is available over the counter. Status asthmaticus Used less often than β_2-selective	¢: Since these cause more side effects

*Rem: The heart is represented by The Phunny Pharm train throughout the Phunny Pharm.

β₂-Selective Agonists in General

BAT PM

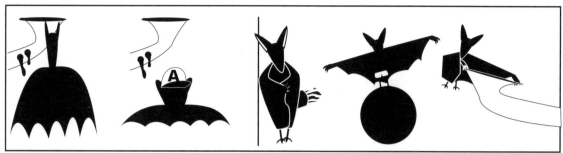

Bitolterol	Albuterol	Terbutaline	Pirbuterol	Metaproterenol

N   All have -ter- in their name and first initials spell <u>BAT PM</u>:
> <u>B</u>itolterol
> <u>A</u>lbuterol
> <u>T</u>erbutaline
>
> <u>P</u>irbuterol
> <u>M</u>etaproterenol

They cause <u>ter</u>ror; and <u>BAT</u>s come out in the <u>PM</u>:

> The <u>tall</u> bat <u>bit</u> the <u>wall</u>.
> <u>Al</u> the bat <u>bit</u> the <u>wall</u>.
> Fast bat ⇒ <u>turbo</u> bat. He <u>leans</u> against the tube wall → enlarge. <u>Turbo</u> <u>bat</u> + <u>lean</u>.
> The <u>p</u>erforming bat, whose <u>butt</u> hit <u>the</u> <u>wall</u>
> The bat who is a <u>pro</u> at <u>tearing</u> the <u>wall</u>

Tox   Limited 2° to limited systemic absorption and selectivity

At higher doses, can get absorption

The bats that fly in the PM prefer to not change into vampires.

When there are too many bats, they will get into the blood and change into a vampire.

<u>Tremor</u>

Can <u>shake</u> from fear of these bats

Rt   Aerosol inhaled

Bats can fly.

Uses   **Symptomatic** relief from asthma

Exercise-induced asthma prophylaxis

¢: From mechanism of action

Corticosteroids in General

The Firefighters

mech   Decrease bronchial hyperreactivity by decreasing <u>inflammation</u>

Inhibits phospholipase A₂ activity, basophil-mediator release, and histamine synthesis (no effect on mast cell release)

Decrease the number of mucosal mast cells

Delayed onset of action

Firefighters extinguish the <u>fire</u> in the lung tubes, thereby preventing the tubes from closing.

The firefighters do not open the tubes directly, they only stop the fire, so it takes time for the tubes to open.

Tox   With systemic therapy: osteoporosis, cataracts, hypertension, appetite stimulation and weight gain.

Uses   Prophylaxis ⇒ better than treatment of symptoms

Firefighters have lookout towers to prevent the fires. This is better than having to call in the bats.

Now considered first-line treatment of asthma

Inhaled is preferred over systemic administration because it will avoid the toxicity.

Systemic Corticosteroids

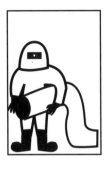

Prednisone and Methylprednisolone

Rt	PO/IV

Enters body through the ocean and walks to the fire with water from the ocean

Uses	Asthma not adequately controlled by bronchodilators and inhaled corticosteroid
	To regain control after exacerbation of asthma
	Generally, try to avoid chronic use because of the associated systemic toxicity.

Inhaled Corticosteroids   Firefighter Pilots

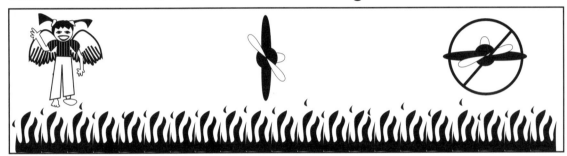

Beclomethasone   Flunisolide   Triamcinolone Acetonide

N	Beclomethasone
	Flunisolide
	Triamcinolone acetonide
Dist	Get minimal systemic absorption unless high dose
Tox	Oral candidiasis if don't rinse mouth with H_2O after use
Rt	Aerosol
Uses	First line for treatment of asthma

Becky is messy in putting out the fire in her zone.
Flew in on his side to put out the fire
Tries to sin alone when he flies
Will not fly into the rest of the Phunny Pharm unless there are a lot of firefighters used
Will leave candy behind in the mouth

Firefighters are pilots and therefore fly.

Methylxanthines

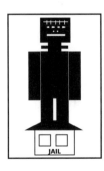

Theophylline   Theo Fills In—Frankenstein

N	Theophylline
mech	Bronchodilation by an uncertain mechanism
Met	Many factors affect metabolism— 95% by liver.
	Inhibit metabolism: older age, liver disease, inhibitors of P-450
	Accelerate metabolism: young age, stimulators of P-450
$t_{1/2}$	Wide variability

Theo Fills In—Frankenstein
He's strong enough to pull air tunnel open.
Police* are after Theo.

¢: Because of all of the things that affect its metabolism

---

*Rem: Police ⇒ liver metabolism.

Tox	Must monitor systemic levels:	
	Abdominal discomfort	
	Seizures	
	Arrhythmias	
	Death	
Rt	PO, IV	Enters body through the ocean and walks to the fire. He is too heavy to fly.
Uses	Nocturnal asthma	Theo Fills In; likes to work at <u>night</u>
	Asthma refractory to β-agonists and inhaled steroids	

Cromolyn

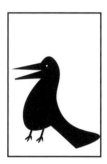

Cromolyn Na

mech	Inhibits mediator release from mast cells
	No bronchodilating effects
Tox	Minimal—generally benign
Rt	<u>Aerosol</u>
Uses	Prophylaxis—especially in allergic asthma

Crow the Raven

The crow flies in and puts out some fires.

The crow has no arms to open the tubes.

The crow is nice.

The crow can <u>fly</u>.

Can help out at the fire lookout

Anticholinergic

Ipratropium

mech	Bronchodilation by inhibition of cholinergic receptors
	Additive effect with β-agonists
Rt	Aerosol inhaled
Uses	First-line treatment in COPD

I Pray to Trap 'em

Prevents the three musketeer cubs from closing down the air tubes

Can work together with the bats

I use my airplane to fly into where the three musketeer cubs live.

Drug Index

2-Chloroethylnitrosureas 67
5-Fluorouracil, 66
5-FU, 66
6-Mercaptopurine, 66
Acebutolol, 103, 169
Acetaminophen, 191
Acetazolamide, 157
Acetylcholine, 79
Actinomycin D, 64
Acyclovir, 58
Adenosine, 171
Adriamycin, 64
Al(OH)$_3$, 195
Albuterol, 98, 201
Alpha-methyldopa, 100
Alprazolam, 108
Amantadine, 60, 120
Amikacin, 33, 40
Amiloride, 159
Aminoglutethimide, 70
Amiodarone, 169
Amitriptyline, 126
Amlodipine, 152
Amobarbital, 111
Amoxicillin, 14
Amphetamine, 94
Amphotericin B, 42
Ampicillin, 14
Amrinone, 163
Ara-C, 66
Aspirin, 180, 188
Astemizole, 197
Atenolol, 103
Atracurium, 88, 142
Atropine, 84, 141
Azithromycin, 30
AZT, 57
Aztreonam, 18
Beclomethasone, 202
Benazepril, 153
Benztropine, 84
Bepridil, 152
Bethanechol, 79
Bitolterol, 98, 201
Bleomycin, 64

Bretylium tosylate, 169
Bromocriptine, 119
Bupivacaine, 144
Bumetanide, 157
Butorphanol, 133
CaCO$_3$, 195
Captopril, 153
Carbachol, 80
Carbamazepine, 114
Carbenicillin, 14
Carbidopa, 118
Carmustine, 68
Cefaclor, 21
Cefadroxil, 20
Cefamandole, 21
Cefazolin, 20
Cefoperazone, 21
Cefotaxime, 21
Cefotetan, 21
Cefoxitin, 21
Ceftazidime, 21
Ceftriaxone, 21
Cefuroxime, 21
Cephalexin, 20
Cephalothin, 20
Chlorambucil, 67
Chloramphenicol, 29
Chlordiazepoxide, 109
Chloroguanide, 47
Chloroquine, 46, 51
Chlorothiazide, 158
Chlorpheniramine, 197
Chlorpromazine, 123
Cholestyramine, 174
Cimetidine, 193
Ciprofloxacin, 36
Cisplatin, 68
Clarithromycin, 30
Clavulanate, 16
Clindamycin, 30
Clofibrate, 175
Clonazepam, 109, 116
Clonidine, 101
Clorazepate, 109
Clotrimazole, 42

Cloxacillin, 13
Clozapine, 124
Codeine, 133
Colestipol, 174
Cromolyn, 198
Cromolyn Na, 203
Cyclopentolate, 85
Cyclophosphamide, 67
Cycloserine, 40
Cytosine arabinoside, 66
d-Tubocurare, 88
Dactinomycin, 64
Daunorubicin, 64
ddI, 59
Demeclocycline, 27
Desipramine, 126
Diazepam, 109, 141
Diazoxide, 150
Dicloxacillin, 13
Dideoxyinosine, 59
Digitalis, 161
Digitoxin, 162
Digoxin, 162
Dihydropyridines, 152
Diloxanide furoate, 51
Diltiazem, 152, 170
Diphenhydramine, 197
Dipyridamole, 181
Disopyramide, 166
Dobutamine, 97, 163
Dopamine, 97, 163
Doxorubicin, 64
Doxycycline, 27
Droperidol, 124, 142
Echothiophate, 81
Edrophonium, 80
Enalapril, 153
Enflurane, 139
Enoxacin, 36
Ephedrine, 94
Epinephrine, 95, 200
Erythromycin, 30
Esmolol, 103, 169
Estrogen, 70
Ethacrynic Acid, 157

Ethambutol, 40
Ethosuximide, 116
Etomidate, 141
Etoposide, 69
Famotidine, 193
Felodipine, 152
Fentanyl, 131, 141
Flecainide, 168
Fluconazole, 42
Flucytosine, 44
Flumazenil, 110
Flunisolide, 202
Fluoxetine, 128
Fluphenazine, 123
Flurazepam, 109
Flutamide, 70
Foscarnet, 61
Fosinopril, 153
Furosemide, 158
Gallamine, 88
Ganciclovir, 58
Gemfibrozil, 175
Gentamicin, 33
Griseofulvin, 43
Haloperidol, 124
Halothane, 139
Heparin, 181
Histamine, 186
Hydralazine, 149
Hydrochlorothiazide, 158
Hydrocodone, 131
Hydromorphone, 131
Ibuprofen, 189
Idoxuridine, 59
Ifosfamide, 67
Imipenem, 17
Imipramine, 126
Indomethacin, 189
Interferons, 60
Ipratropium, 85, 203
Isocarboxazid, 127
Isoetharine, 96, 200
Isoflurane, 139
Isoflurophate, 81
Isoniazid, 39
Isoproterenol, 96, 200
Isosorbide dinitrate, 150
Isoxazoles, 14
Isradipine, 152
Itraconazole, 42
Kanamycin, 34
Ketamine, 140
Ketoconazole, 42
Ketorolac, 190
L-Dopa, 118

Labetalol, 101
Lansoprazole, 194
Leukotrienes, 185
Leuprolide, 70
Lidocaine, 144, 167
Lincomycin, 30
Lisinopril, 153
Lithium, 129
Lomefloxacin, 36
Lomustine, 68
Loperamide, 132
Loratadine, 197
Lorazepam, 108
Losartan, 154
Lovastatin, 174
Mannitol, 157
Mebendazole, 52
Mechlorethamine, 67
Meclofenamate, 189
Mefloquine, 47
Meperidine, 131
Mephenteramine, 94
Metaproterenol, 98, 201
Methacholine, 80
Methacycline, 27
Methadone, 131
Methamphetamine, 94
Methenamine, 37
Methacillin, 13
Methohexital, 111, 140
Methotrexate, 65
Methoxyflurane, 139
Methylnitrosurea 67
Methylprednisolone, 202
Metoprolol, 103
Metrifonate 56
Metronidazole, 51
Mexiletine, 167
Mezlocillin, 14
Miconazole, 42
Midazolam, 108, 141
Milrinone, 163
Minocycline, 27
Minoxidil, 149
Misoprostol, 195
Moricizine, 166
Morphine, 131, 141
Nadolol, 102
Nafcillin, 13
NaHCO$_3$, 195
Nalbuphine, 133
Nalidixic acid, 35
Naloxone, 133
Naproxen, 189
Neomycin, 34

Neostigmine, 80
Netilmicin, 34
Nicardipine, 152
Nicotinic acid, 174
Nifedipine, 152
Nitrofurantoin, 37
Nitroglycerine, 150
Nitrous oxide, 138
Nizatidine, 193
Norepinephrine, 96
Norfloxacin, 36
Nortriptyline, 126
Nystatin, 42
Ofloxacin, 36
Omeprazole, 194
Oxacillin, 13
Oxazepam, 108
Oxycodone, 131
p-Aminosalicylic acid, 40
Pancuronium, 88, 142
Penicillin G, 13
Penicillin V, 13
Pentazocine, 133
Pentobarbital, 111
Phenelzine, 127
Phenobarbital, 112, 115
Phenoxybenzamine, 101
Phentolamine, 101
Phenylbutazone, 189
Phenylephrine, 96
Phenytoin, 114, 167
Physostigmine, 80
Pilocarpine, 80
Pindolol, 102
Piperacillin, 14
Pirbuterol, 98, 201
Pirenzepine, 91
Piroxicam, 189
Polymyxin B, 31
Potassium iodide, 44
Pralidoxime, 82
Pravastin, 174
Praziquantel, 52
Prazosin, 102
Prednisone, 202
Primaquine, 46
Primidone, 116
Probenicid, 16
Probucol, 176
Procainamide, 166
Procaine, 144
Prochlorperazine, 123
Propafenone, 168
Propantheline, 86
Propoxyphene, 132

Propranolol, 102, 169
Prostaglandins, 185
Pyrantel, 52
Pyrazinamide, 40
Pyridostigmine, 80
Pyrilamine, 197
Pyrimethamine, 47
Quinapril, 153
Quinidine, 166
Quinine, 47
Ramipril, 153
Ranitidine, 193
Reserpine, 100
Ribavirin, 58
Rifampin, 39
Rimantadine, 60
Risperidone, 124
Scopolamine, 84, 141
Secobarbital, 111
Selegiline, 119
Sertraline, 128
Silver sulfadiazine, 25
Simvastatin, 174
Sodium nitroprusside, 150
Sodium stibogluconate, 51
Sotalol, 171
Spectinomycin, 31
Spironolactone, 159
Streptokinase, 183
Streptomycin, 34, 40

Streptozotocin, 68
Succinylcholine, 89, 142
Sucralfate, 184
Sufentanil, 131
Sulbactam, 16
Sulfacetamide, 25
Sulfadiazine, 24
Sulfamerazine, 24
Sulfamethazine, 24
Sulfamethoxazole, 24
Sulfinpyrazone, 180
Sulfisoxazole, 24
Sulfonamides, 47
Sulfones, 47
Sulindac, 189
Tamoxifen, 70
Taxol, 69
Tazobactam, 16
Temazepam, 108
Terazosin, 102
Terbutaline, 98, 201
Terfenadine, 197
Tetracycline, 27
Theophylline, 202
Thiopental, 111, 140
Thioridazine, 123
Thiothixine, 123
Ticarcillin, 14
Ticlopidine, 181
Timolol, 102

Tissue plasminogen activator, 183
Tobramycin, 33
Tocainide, 167
Tolmetin, 189
TPA, 183
Tramadol, 191
Tranylcypromine, 127
Trazodone, 129
Triamcinolone acetonide, 202
Triamterine, 159
Triazolam, 108
Trifluoperazine, 123
Trihexyphenidyl, 119
Trimethaphan, 86, 150
Trimethoprim, 25
Triple sulfas, 24
Tropicamide, 85
Tyramine, 95
Urokinase, 183
Valproate, 115
Vancomycin, 17
Vecuronium, 88, 142
Verapamil, 152, 170
Vidarabine, 59
Vinblastine, 69
Vincristine, 69
VP16–213, 69
Warfarin, 182
Zidovudine (AZT), 59